Laboratory Science and M

An introduction

Maxine Lintern

Director, PG Certificate in Teaching and Learning in Higher Education
Lecturer in Medical Science
University of Birmingham

Foreword by
Baroness Susan Greenfield

Radcliffe Publishing
Oxford • Seattle

Radcliffe Publishing Ltd
18 Marcham Road
Abingdon
Oxon OX14 1AA
United Kingdom

www.radcliffe-oxford.com
Electronic catalogue and worldwide online ordering facility.

_____

New research and clinical experience can result in changes in treatment and drug therapy. Readers of this book should therefore check the most recent product information on any drug they may prescribe to ensure they are complying with the manufacturer's recommendations concerning dosage, the method and duration of administration, and contraindications. Neither the publisher nor the authors accept liability for any injury or damage arising from this publication.

British Library Cataloguing in Publication Data

A catalogue record for this book is available from the British Library.

ISBN-10: 1 84619 016 9
ISBN-13: 978 1 84619 016 2

Typeset by Anne Joshua & Associates, Oxford
Printed and bound by TJ International Ltd, Padstow, Cornwall

Contents

Foreword

When I first started in a laboratory, an alarming 33 years ago, I had no idea of the world into which I was entering. I still remember the bewildering differences in expectations from my normal life: standards of cleanliness, of accuracy and of safety – these were all very different from my experience, even in laboratories at school. At that time science lessons, even in the sixth form, involved trooping in en masse, and having experiments laid out before you with an instruction sheet that would also indicate what results you were to expect. I fear that even at the university level many practical classes were along similar lines. Only when I started in a research laboratory as a graduate student did I encounter the shock of needing to use one's initiative but, at the same time, not having a ready source of information to do so.

For whilst teaching laboratories are arguably extensions of a classroom, research laboratories most emphatically are not. Here things move at a very fast pace, decisions have to be made very quickly, and there is not necessarily a consensus or obvious way forward: moreover, one cannot assume that, even for a relatively junior member of the lab, there will be someone to whom you can speak immediately. And there is so much to bear in mind: before everything there is health and safety, which goes way beyond mere common-sense. There are also new concepts to bear in mind: how to prepare solutions and prepare experiments: however well-taught one may be, it is very rare that you have actually had to design and set up an experiment from scratch!

Then there is a whole range of new sophisticated and expensive techniques that will not necessarily have featured in either school or university science education. Understanding the basic concepts, as well as the procedures, is far from trivial and far from obvious, and once one is conducting an experiment, the interpretation of data, again, requires skill and knowledge.

In order to make the most of one's laboratory experience and to enjoy designing, conducting and interpreting experiments, this book is long overdue. Compared to 30 years ago, there are now ever increasingly stricter regulations in place, whilst techniques are increasingly refined with sophisticated and expensive equipment. It may not be possible to find the right person at the right time to answer a query, but this book, on the other hand, can always be with you – it will enable you to prepare as much as possible, and reduce the risk of you being caught short in a crisis, or with a problem that requires an instant and key decision. It will give you the marvellous opportunity, that I never had, of knowing what to expect when you start in a laboratory. But it is not just a one-off read, it will also be your constant companion whilst you are in the laboratory – always there with the correct answer when your colleagues either don't know, or are too busy to give you the time that you need.

I only wish such a book had been available to me when I first started research, as it would have saved me and avoided many tears, upsets, and wastage of time and money, not to mention, on certain occasions, possible health risks. Spanning as it does the procedural through to the basic concepts, details of the latest techniques, as well as ethical considerations, and advice on presenting data, this book covers the whole gamut of expertise that will equip you for a productive and exciting life in science and medicine research.

Baroness Susan Greenfield CBE

October 2006

Preface

I have had many bright, capable undergraduate and postgraduate science and medical students come into my lab to begin research projects, full of theoretical knowledge, but with no real idea of the practicalities of life in the lab. As a consequence I used to spend quite a while trying to identify their needs, finding them to be (usually) more or less the same each year. These included a lack of understanding of how basic chemical concepts are used in the lab, difficulty in manipulating common units, problems with recording, processing and data etc. This prompted me to produce a small handout of basic lab skills, to help get them up to speed in a shorter space of time, therefore maximising their productive lab time. This short handout developed into Section 1 of this book.

They also sometimes muddled different research techniques, and so I thought a quick overview of some common methods would be useful, to help them to understand what was going on around them in the lab, and in the papers that they were reading.

With this basic coverage of many biomedical techniques as well as underlying scientific concepts, the overview grew into Section 2 of this book. Together the two sections aim to impart my experience and that of my colleagues, of working day-to-day in a lab environment to new researchers, to help them on the road to interesting and useful results.

Maxine Lintern
October 2006

About the author

Dr Maxine Lintern has been a biomedical researcher and lecturer in medical science for many years. She has supervised numerous under-graduate and postgraduate science and medical students through their research projects. Currently she is working in staff development at the University of Birmingham as Director of the PGCert in Teaching and Learning in Higher Education, engaging with lecturing staff as they develop their teaching practice in all subject areas. She is also an associate member of the School of Biosciences, and a Fellow of the Higher Education Academy. Her research interests include the plasticity of the cholinergic synapse and the development of laboratory teaching practice.

Acknowledgements

My grateful thanks are extended to:

- Dr Angelo Agathanggelou (my wonderful husband) who made major contributions to Chapters 8, 9 and 10 as well as providing some of the pretty pictures of cells!
- my colleagues, past and present – especially Mrs Debbie Ruston and Dr Anna Rowe for comments and useful criticisms (and pictures!), and Professor Margaret Smith for teaching me how to be a researcher in the first place!
- Professor David Morton for advice and useful criticism of Chapter 11
- staff of the UB Health and Safety Unit, for their help with the research for Chapter 2
- my students for inspiring me to write this book in the first place, in the hope that it will help future science and medical students in their research careers.

Dedication

This book is dedicated to my family: Angelo, Alexander, Joshua and Elizabeth who have supported me throughout, even when I was working late (again) or hassling them for their contributions, and my parents for their continued love and support.

List of boxes, tables and figures

Abbreviations

ACDP	Advisory Committee on Dangerous Pathogens
amu	atomic mass unit
AP	alkaline phosphatase
ATCC	American Type Culture Collection
CGAP	Cancer Genome Anatomy Project
CGH	comparative genomic hybridisation
COSHH	control of substances hazardous to health
DAPI	4′,6-diamidino-2-phenylindole
DEPC	diethylpyrocarbonate
DMEM	Dulbecco's Modified Eagle's Medium
dNTP	deoxyribonucleotide triphosphate
EBV	Epstein–Barr virus
ELISA	enzyme-linked immunosorbent assay
ExPASY	Expert Protein Analysis System
FCS	fetal calf serum
FITC	fluorescein isothiocyanate
FW	formula weight
HCG	human chorionic gonadotrophin
HEK	human embryonic kidney (cells)
HeLa	Henrietta Lacks (cells)
HRP	horseradish peroxidase
HSE	Health and Safety Executive
HUVEC	human umbilical venous epithelial cell
IgA	immunoglobulin A
IgG	immunoglobulin G
IgM	immunoglobulin M
MEF	mouse embryonal fibroblast
MW	molecular weight
NACWO	named animal care and welfare officer
NCBI	National Center for Biotechnology Information
OMIM	Online Mendelian Inheritance in Man
ORF	open reading frame
PAGE	polyacrylamide gel electrophoresis
PCR	polymerase chain reaction
PDA	personal digital assistant

RFM	relative formula mass
RT	reverse transcriptase
RT-PCR	reverse transcription PCR
SDS	sodium dodecyl sulphate
SI	Système International (units)
siRNA	small inhibitory RNA
SOP	standard operating procedures

Chapter 1

Introduction

What this book is about

Scientific research is a voyage of discovery, a journey through the murkier corners of the unknown towards the lofty goal of enlightenment and understanding. There is nothing more rewarding than actually discovering something that no-one knew before, and adding it to the sum of human knowledge. For philosophers and theoretical physicists this may be achieved by sitting around thinking deeply (while perhaps drinking copious amounts of herbal tea or strong coffee respectively!). For biomedical scientists however, it means actually getting your lab coat on and getting your hands dirty.

If you are about to embark on your first experience of real lab work, it may well be a rather daunting prospect, and you might be wondering what to expect. You will probably spend the first few days trying to find your feet, the toilet and the kettle; let alone whatever it is that you are supposed to do! This book is designed to give you, the new researcher, practical hands-on advice to help you get started with your research, and it should be of use throughout your time working in a research lab. It is full of useful equations, calculations, tips and advice to help your research project run smoothly, and for you (and your supervisor/colleagues) to get the most out of it. It contains a range of concepts from basic chemical principles, which you may have forgotten you knew, to sexy new molecular biology techniques. Each topic is covered in a general way for the non-expert, to give you a feel for the technique and to provide enough background knowledge for you to be able to decide if it is something that you might want/need to use in the future. At the very least it should help you to follow your colleagues' presentations!

As well as the science, working in research also requires you to acquire and develop some of those ever-useful and totally fundamental transferable skills – organisation, independence, initiative and determination. You will also begin to appreciate the difference between listening to dry facts in a cold lecture theatre, and practical enquiry-based learning, working at the bench alongside a leader in the field. In research no two days are the same; sudden disasters and set backs can be followed by almost perfect experiments and ideal results. There are highs and lows, frantic days and tedious days, complete frustration when things just don't go your way, followed by jubilation when it all comes together and you have a success. Some of you (undergraduates) may be considering a career in science and you may have already started your feet along that pathway. This book can help you make the transition from an inexperienced 'student' with factual knowledge and conceptual understanding, but with little experience or confidence with application, to a competent, confident researcher on their way to an interesting result and a solid publication. The remit of the following chapters is deliberately broad to give you a feel for as many topics as possible. However, where appropriate there is support and suggestions to help you find out further information, for example books, protocols, web pages etc. In this way the handbook can act as a springboard to launch your understanding of real biomedical research, and with it your career.

Who should read this book

This book is aimed at anyone who is about to embark, or has recently embarked on a research project within a working laboratory, at undergraduate, postgraduate or early post-doctoral level. The subject focus is quite wide, encompassing biomedical science/biochemistry/medical research and molecular biology. If you are an undergraduate starting a final year research project, an intercalating medical student undertaking a science degree, a new PhD student or trainee research technician, then this book is for you! Practising medics coming back into a laboratory situation will also find a lot of useful information here which will help to guide them through the pitfalls of re-entering the research domain.

However this list is not exclusive, as much of the information will also be useful to more experienced researchers such as contract research staff, post-docs and beyond, especially as a refresher or quick reference guide. Very keen undergraduates will also find a lot of information here, which will help you to prepare for future practical classes and research projects, and to reinforce your understanding of key concepts. All of the content can be used as a stepping-stone to discover more detailed information.

Why you need this book

If you want to arrive on the first day in a new lab and look good, then when your supervisor says 'go and make up this buffer to 0.2 mM and use it to make a serial dilution of this new expensive drug we want to test . . .', you want to be able to say 'OK, point me to the pipettes'. If the post-doc says 'you need to fill out all these COSHH forms first', this book will help you to understand what is required. If the grad student says 'are you doing ELISAs or westerns?', you need to be able to discuss the differences. When you are asked to write up your experimental data for a lab meeting, you need to know the best format to use.

Becoming a good biomedical researcher, like everything else in life, doesn't just happen overnight. Exploring your knowledge and skills base, and the gaps therein allows you to develop your approach to research in a systematic and productive manner. By taking advantage of the experience bundled into this volume, you are giving yourself the advantage of both increased factual knowledge and useful practical applications which will help you on the road to achieving your goals, whether that is a good first degree, your first publication, that first grant or a Nobel prize!

If you want to give yourself a flying start in your lab career, then this book is for you.

How to use this book

This book is arranged in two sections. The first section deals with basic, but important underlying concepts such as health and safety, and how to calculate concentrations for making up reagents and handle your data. This includes some equations, which are repeated in the 'Formulae at a glance' chapter at the end of the book. It also gives you ideas and advice about how to *do* your research; such as how to plan experiments and how to keep track of your results and data. Chapter 6 deals with the sometimes mysterious concept of scientific writing, and offers practical approaches to effectively communicate your amazing results to the world.

Section 2 looks more specifically at some common techniques and experimental approaches found in biomedical research laboratories, although the list is, of course, not exhaustive! Each technique is briefly described to give you a feel for it, and enough understanding to appreciate its application and uses. It should also help you to understand a little better the research papers you may (*should*) be reading. The protocols given are very general, and not intended to be used directly in the lab!

Rather you should use them as foundation knowledge and as a starting point to kick off your further investigations. If you decide to use one of these approaches you will need to obtain much more specific protocols, from the literature or specific lab manuals, but hopefully the more detailed information in the protocols will be easier to understand and implement once you have fully grasped the basic principles.

Many of the references used in this book are web based. This is a deliberate policy as they can guide you to useful and interesting sources of further information that you can immediately follow up. As we all know web pages are not usually peer reviewed, and the scientific data on them cannot always be relied upon, so always be careful how you use them. They are also very rarely permanent fixtures and so it may be that though the links were sound at the time of writing, they have moved by the time you come to look at them. Hopefully with a little digging and net searching you should be able to find the strays or their replacements, and then can let us know!

In the discussions of particular techniques or approaches, occasionally particular commercial products have been mentioned. This is in no way an endorsement of the quality, reliability or appropriateness of those particular products. Rather they are only being mentioned as an example of the type of items available from the plethora of biomedical suppliers. It is strongly recommended that you always shop around for anything you are considering spending your hard-earned grant money on!

I hope that you will find this book useful, and that it will become tatty, dog-eared and stained from spending its time stuffed in your lab coat pocket and out on the lab bench. I hope that it becomes your first source of reference as you begin your career in the lab as a biomedical researcher, and that it remains useful as your experience increases. In short I hope that the first steps that you take towards the next biomedical break-through are helped, supported and inspired by the information contained in this book.

Section 1

Basic concepts

Chapter 2

Health and safety in the laboratory

Safety in the laboratory

Labs are undoubtedly dangerous places. In most laboratories, where you will be working on your research project there will be compounds, chemicals, organisms and equipment that could cause you serious harm or even death. Make no mistake – people have been seriously injured or have even died in laboratory accidents, and even minor mishaps can have a negative influence on your work and research output.

Safety is therefore a very serious issue and should underlie everything that you do in the laboratory. It is *your* responsibility to make sure that you understand fully all of the hazards involved in your work, and those of the people working around you. Ignorance is no protection from either harm or responsibility!

Every lab poses different hazards to the inexperienced researcher, depending on the nature of the work that is being undertaken there. Specific hazards such as radioactive materials are subject to very strict guidelines, and will be addressed later in this chapter. However some concepts are fairly generic in so far as they can be applied to all laboratory work and should form the basis of your personal safety working code.

The idea of a personal code of practice illustrates that you have engaged fully with the general, local and specific guidelines for your work. It is something that you should spend time considering seriously with respect to the kind of work you are doing and the type of lab you are working in.

Box 2.1   General health and safety guidelines

- No unprofessional behaviour of any kind – this includes rushing around, throwing things.
- No eating or drinking of any kind in the lab.
- Lab coats should be worn while working in the lab, but removed on exit.

(continued)

- Gloves and other protective equipment should be worn when appropriate and discarded in the correct place when leaving the lab.
- Hands should always be washed as you leave the lab – usually there will be a 'hand wash only' sink for this purpose.
- Any sharps such as needles, scalpels, pipette tips etc must be disposed of into the 'sharps bin'.
- Usually biologically contaminated waste is discarded into 'bio-hazard' labelled yellow bags, while normal rubbish goes into black bags – check for the local regulations in your lab.
- All accidents must be reported to your supervisor, lab manager, and probably the safety officer for the department/division.
- Students are not usually allowed to be in the labs unsupervised or out of hours (e.g. late at night or on weekends).
- You should always try to work in a clean and tidy manner – accidents are more likely if you are working in a mess.
- Label everything you use with your name, date, compound or sample, concentration and the associated hazard.
- Be aware of the hazard symbols and what they mean.
- Specific hazards such as radioactive materials, pathogens etc require additional care and are subject to further regulations such as wearing radioactive monitoring badges, training courses and confinement to designated areas or rooms.

Common hazard symbols

Hazard symbols are visual signs usually seen on the outside of containers, which show you what hazard is associated with the contents. They are pictorial, and so even if you cannot read the associated text, you still have a fair idea of the risks. For instance, the skull and crossed bones representing 'toxic' is an unmistakable warning of the possibility of death if consumed!

However you should make sure that you take time to study and learn the full meanings of the symbols, and what precautions need to be in place before you begin to handle substances with those hazards (*see* Figure 2.1 (*see* plate section)).

COSHH and risk assessment

Understanding the nature of the hazard of a particular compound is not enough. The amount/concentration of the compound and the type of potential exposure is also very important. A common chemical such as salt (NaCl) may seem innocuous enough; after all we all use it in our kitchens! However mix a strong enough solution and drink it, and it becomes a poison. Similarly, extremely toxic compounds can be used in the laboratory setting safely because they are handled in very low quantities or concentrations. Thus the relative risk of hurt is related not only to the compound itself, but just as importantly to the *way* in which it is used.

For every laboratory procedure, and every chemical used in that procedure, a 'risk assessment' must be compiled. This is a paper study looking at what chemical is used, in what procedure, and under what precautionary measures. Thus keeping to low concentrations and using appropriate protection such as a lab coat, gloves and eye protectors reduces the danger of using a toxic chemical; and this is reflected in the risk assessment. Procedures in an established lab will have already been assessed in this way, and guidelines or 'standard operating procedures' will have been drawn up. You must make yourself familiar with them for every procedure that you undertake, and new risk assessments should be compiled for every new procedure you may introduce during the course of your research. You should also have an awareness of the procedures being used by your colleagues in the lab. This effectively means being aware of the potential hazards on the lab bench next to you!

Important information about *how* that chemical is or may become dangerous is also included in the assessment. For example, a compound that produces toxic fumes would need to be handled exclusively in a fume hood of appropriate rating; a skin absorbable poison would be handled wearing special gloves. Most compounds also have a 'LD_{50}' to guide you. This is a statement of how much of this compound was required to give a 'lethal dose' to half a cohort of (usually) rats. LD_{50} data can show relative risks between compounds, and human LD_{50} information is available for some compounds. Pharmaceutical companies produce similar data for drugs and medicines.

All of this information can help you to modify your working environment and your behaviour in that environment appropriately to ensure best safe practice, and reduce the chances of accidents occurring. This is formalised in the UK by the COSHH regulations. This stands for control of substances hazardous to health. The Health and Safety Executive (HSE) are the government body responsible for producing guidelines and legislation, and are a very good source of information when thinking about risk assessments. Institutions usually have their own health and safety department or unit who will produce local guidelines and regulations and help with the production of risk assessments and standard operating procedures.

Risk assessment can be approached in more than one way. You may decide to work systematically, looking at each different activity routinely and occasionally performed in the lab environment, or you may look at certain groups of hazards such as chemical substances, machinery, electrical items etc. Another approach is to work geographically i.e. room-to-room, lab-to-lab. However you organise your approach there are five main steps to work through:[1]

- identify what the hazard is
- identify who potentially may be affected by that hazard
- ascertain what the risks arising from that hazard are, and make decisions and policies to control and reduce those risks
- set those policies and practices into protocols or standard operating procedures (SOP)
- record the information in a standardised and easily accessible manner.

Chemical hazards

When working with different chemical substances, and assessing the relative hazards and risks, there are a range of criteria that affect the final assessment. Identifying and regulating chemical hazards is *not* simply producing a list of the possible hazards of a particular chemical or a collection of safety data sheets! This type of information, while a useful starting point or source of reference, is not enough to allow you to make decisions about the way you handle a particular chemical.

Firstly you must understand the form of the substance; is it gas, liquid, powder or fume etc? You must also be aware that a particular substance may change its form during the course of normal handling e.g. water past $100°C$ turns into a gas, and so the nature of the hazard changes. Physical properties such as boiling or melting point are very important, as is information on stability or reactivity with other compounds. This basic information can easily be found on the manufacturer data sheets, catalogues and often on the side of the container. Similarly, most containers will have a hazard label covering the main hazards as previously described, e.g. toxic or corrosive. Additional labelling may also include phrases such as 'may cause cancer' or 'flammable in air'. This is really only the start of your understanding of the risk of the hazard to you or other workers' health. You also need to know if the risk is acute – a single contact can cause serious effects; chronic – repeated contacts may cause an effect; additive – damages health if mixed with something else or with consecutive exposures, or if there are both short- and long-term potential effects to consider. Other phrases that you may come across which it may be useful to define here are shown in Box 2.2.

Box 2.2   'Hazard' phrases

- *Allergenic*: may cause hypersensitivity
- *Carcinogenic*: may cause cancer
- *Mutagenic*: may change genetic material (DNA) affecting the inherited characteristics
- *Reproductive*: may impair or damage fertility
- *Teratogenic*: may cause damage to an embryo

Secondly, what you are doing with the chemical has a major impact on the potential risk. The amount of the chemical used, whether different chemicals are going to be mixed and in what way, all must be considered. Other conditions such as temperature or pressure, reliance on protective equipment, containment etc should also be considered. You must not forget to take into account what could go wrong, if mistakes are made or if equipment fails.

Next you must consider how a particular chemical substance could potentially cause harm by coming into contact with your body. Routes include inhalation, swallowing, absorption through the eyes or the skin, contact damage to either the eyes or the skin, and injection into the body by contaminated sharp objects or equipment such as hypodermic needles. Understanding this will help you to decide on the correct protective measures such as gloves, goggles or only using that chemical in a fume cupboard. Sometimes the substance itself creates a hazardous situation because of its effects on the environment. For example the sudden release of a non-toxic gas such as nitrogen may deplete the percentage of available oxygen in the room. The risk of fire or explosion must also be considered; does the compound easily catch fire if there is a source of ignition or is it so unstable it can spontaneously explode? Other factors to consider are incompatible mixes such as chemicals that react on contact with air or water. The frequency of using a particular chemical may also impact on your decisions; a very occasional use of a chemical is less of a potential risk than if you have to handle it every day.

The people who may be affected by the chemical are your next consideration. This obviously includes the researchers performing the experiment or procedure, but you must also think about the people on the other side of the lab; are they potentially at risk? What about other less obvious staff such as office staff, cleaners or security guards? They may be only passing through your lab (often when you yourself are not around), but are you considering your hazards in light of their potential presence, and possible lack of familiarity with the chemicals you are using?

All of this information, once properly collated, can help you to prevent or control the risk as much as possible. This includes, as previously stated, using correct labelling, choosing the appropriate protective equipment, good standards of chemical practice etc, and will help you to identify the need for any additional information or training. Once this procedure is in place you cannot just forget about it! Your hazard/risk assessment must have built into it some flexibility for changing circumstances and an ongoing monitoring procedure. This should include a periodic review addressing issues such as: are the procedures working adequately, is the equipment being properly maintained, has anything changed to make the current procedures inadequate? In addition, have you considered what emergency measures you would need in a worst-case scenario? What first aid procedures/facilities do you need, what contamination risks would there be to the workplace or the environment?

This is a lot of information to think about, but it is very important that you get it right; your life might very well depend on it! The ideas and concepts covered in this section are not the full story; they are merely a brief overview to help give you some perspective on the subject. When undertaking any kind of risk/hazard assessment it is important that you get sound advice and practical help from your institution's health and safety unit or equivalent. They will have lots of experience and probably will have experts in particular areas that can help you to make your assessment a positive, constructive procedure, and not just a bit of useless bureaucracy that you go through the motions of, and then forget. Some hazards such as biological or radiation need separate additional consideration, and so are discussed in more detail in further sections.

Some useful reference sources in the UK can be found on the HMSO website.[2–4]

Biological hazards

In addition to the considerations discussed in the previous section, there are many additional aspects to the safe usage of biological materials which may potentially pose a health and safety risk. The definition of a biological material in this context is:

> any micro-organism, cell culture, parasite, human or animal tissue (including blood, urine and other body products) or plant materials, which may cause infection, allergy, toxicity or other risks to human health or cause a risk to the environment.[5]

This obviously applies to an awful lot of the stuff that is generally used in a biomedical research lab, and so this particular aspect of health and safety may well be especially pertinent to your situation. For most institutions, although the details will vary from place to place, a general policy of consultation will be enforced. This means that *before* any work commences using biologically hazardous material, the risk assessment is performed and procedures to minimise the risk are put into place. This includes considerations such as the transport and storage of such items, and the emergency procedures and medical support should the worst ever happen. Again everyone involved with the work must understand the risks and the procedures and work with the health and safety at institutional and, if necessary, national levels.

Biological materials are divided into categories depending on how nasty they are, and the rules and regulations differ as you go from 1–4. The HSE Advisory Committee on Dangerous Pathogens (ACDP) makes the decision as to which category each agent falls into, and further information about this body and the list of agents is available from the website.[6]

Only agents in the higher groups 2, 3 and 4 are listed. Examples include Clostridium, Botulinum and Epstein–Barr virus in category 2, yellow fever virus, rabies and HIV in category 3, while category 4 includes Ebola and Lassa fever. For any work involving materials in category 2 or above, formal approval of the project must be obtained from the institution's health and safety, and sometimes the national HSE, which includes checks to ensure that the facilities are up to the required standard, that the people involved are fully trained, and that all the correct handling procedures are present.

Another group of potentially hazardous biological materials that you might find yourself working with are genetically modified organisms. These too are categorised into classes 1–4, which attract different standards of regulations from the departmental/institutional to the national level. Thus, for whatever material you are working with, there is a great deal of institutional and national support to help you to achieve your aims of good results, while working in the safest possible way. It is always in your best interest to work within this framework, and depending on the category level may well be a legal requirement. At the risk of being repetitive, it is important to say again that when you join a new lab, this type of legislation and working practice/procedure will almost certainly already be in place; but you must make sure that you fully familiarise yourself with them, and receive adequate training before you start handling this type of material.

A final consideration is the unfortunate prospect of external persons getting access to, gaining possession of, and then using your dangerous biological materials, possibly in a terrorism situation. In order to counter this possibility, the types of material thought most likely to be at risk from this type of abuse are subject to further regulations. These include notification of the Home Office (in the UK) of the acquisition and usage of these materials. Additional controls regarding storage, security arrangements and accessibility are also enforced, and are subject to inspection by the police authorities. Substances that come into this category include many high-category viruses like Ebola, bacteria such as types of Salmonella and Bacillus anthracis, and toxins like ricin and tetrodotoxin. If your research uses these pathogens/toxins then you must comply with the regulations under the Anti-terrorism, Crime and Security Act (2001).[7] If you were wondering why a particular fridge had a large padlock on it, which only the team leader had a key for, this might be why!

The bottom line for understanding and complying with all of these regulations is taking appropriate advice and always acting under consultation. Many departments/schools have dedicated persons acting as biological safety officers or equivalents who are very experienced in this area, and will be able to help you meet all the requirements you need for the type of work you are doing and handling the types of material you are using.

Radiation hazards

Radiation hazards in labs are usually of the ionising form, and can cause serious adverse biological effects depending on the type of radiation, the energy levels and the length of exposure. Care should be taken to minimise or eliminate the associated risks by adhering to the strict guidelines laid down by the HSE and the institution.[8]

For a researcher to use radioactive substances they must first undergo appropriate training and reach designated levels of competence, and then ensure that they work strictly within the local regulatory guidelines. Most laboratories or departments will have a designated safety officer to over-see use of radioactive substances and ensure good practice. You (and/or your supervisor) are responsible for finding out about the local regula-tions and getting yourself trained.

Common guidelines include restricting work with radioactive sub-stances to a designated and clearly labelled area of the lab. In larger labs this may be a completely separate room (often nicknamed the 'hot' room). Only people who have undergone the correct training and are wearing monitoring badges are allowed to work in this area/room. Every container that comes into contact with a radioactive substance must be clearly labelled with the radioactive warning symbol. All radioactive substances must be closely monitored for usage, and detailed records kept regarding what has come into the lab, how it has been used and how it has been disposed of. There are legal limits controlling the disposal of radioactive substances into the drains or out with 'normal' rubbish, and you must show that you are adhering to this by accounting for every Curie or Becquerel! This will also improve the reliability of the data that you produce, as any level of contamination can obscure or even ruin your results!

The designated areas must also be monitored for any contamination or spillages. The person responsible for overseeing the radioactive usage in your area may perform this routinely, or there may be a lab rota, but it is good practice for you to monitor the working area before you start to work and again when you finish. Thus any 'hot spots' can be quickly deconta-minated, which will help to reduce your exposure and prevent spreading the contamination any further.

Appropriate protective clothing should be worn at all times when handling radioactive substances. This may include a designated lab coat, gloves and possibly eye protection. Monitoring badges, which assess the level of exposure an individual has received, are usually compulsory. It may be that even if you personally are not working with a radioactive substance, but other people in your lab vicinity are, then you will need to have a monitoring badge also. These are usually changed monthly and analysed for exposure levels. Again it is imperative that you are familiar with, and are adhering to, the local regulations in your lab/institution, and the particular hazard working protocol associated with the substances you are using. For example working with 'hot' powders or crystalline compounds has different associated hazards from working with 'hot' liquids!

Hazardous waste

All this hard work with toxic/pathogenic/radioactive material will inevitably lead to the production of waste products. As you would expect, these too are subject to strict rules and regulations to ensure that nothing nasty ends up where it could harm people or the environment. In order to dispose of the waste correctly you must be able to clearly assess what kind of waste it is, and then you can choose the appropriate procedure to follow. Most biomedical labs will have multiple disposal bins, often using a bag colour-coding system. Thus 'ordinary' waste, such as paper, will be disposed of into normal black bags and will be taken away as household/office-type waste. This is handled by cleaning staff, refuse collectors etc, and often ends up on landfill sites which is something to bear in mind when deciding whether something should go in or not.[9]

If waste is considered hazardous as defined by the regulations, then it is subject to greater controls and must be disposed of in a particular way. It is the user's responsibility to decide what form any waste produced is, i.e. the producer of the waste, which means you, does the classification. This will include making sure the correct waste codes are assigned and the correct sealed labelled containers are used. Usually a set of labs or a department will have these arrangements already set up and will have centralised systems for collecting and disposing of things like yellow biohazard bags, animal products/carcasses, sharps containers, radioactive waste for decontamination, halogenated solvents etc. Again, advice and support will be available to help you plan to deal appropriately with the waste you produce, and if in doubt always check. Obviously putting used pipette tips into plastic bags could cause a hazard as they can puncture the bag easily and may stick into someone's skin!

A final word on health and safety

This section on health and safety does not cover all of the potential hazards of working in a laboratory but hopefully will have given you some insight into the way the system works. The take-home message for all aspects of health and safety, using chemicals, biological agents and equipment is to:

- make sure you understand the hazard
- make sure you receive the correct training/instruction on how to use that material in such a way as to minimise any risks to you and your surroundings

- make sure you are fully informed of, and strictly adhere to the policy and legislation around health and safety issues, which apply to you, and the environment you are working in
- always err on the side of caution, and if in doubt, ask!

References

1 *University of Birmingham Health and Safety Guidance – Risk Assessment.* Guidance/17/RA/00.
2 Office of Public Sector Information. www.legislation.hmso.gov.uk (accessed 22 June 2006).
3 Health and Safety Executive Homepage. www.hse.gov.uk (accessed 22 June 2006).
4 *University of Birmingham Health and Safety Guidance – Chemical Hazard and Risk Assessment.* Guidance/22/CHRA/03.
5 *University of Birmingham Health and Safety Policy – Biological Safety.* UHSP/9/BS/05.
6 *Advisory Committee on Dangerous Pathogens – The Approval List of Biological Agents.* www.hse.gov.uk/aboutus/meetings/acdp/index.htm (accessed 22 June 2006).
7 Anti-terrorism, Crime and Security Act (2001). www.opsi.gov.uk/si/si2002/20021558.htm
8 *University of Birmingham Health and Safety Guidance – Use of Ionising Radiation.* Guidance/19/UIR/04.
9 *University of Birmingham Health and Safety Guidance – Hazardous Waste*: *guidance on assessment.* Guidance/11/HWGA/05.

Chapter 3

Underlying chemical concepts

Units

Weights and measures are defined by the agreed Système International and are usually referred to as SI units. The units you will most likely meet in a biological laboratory are mass in grams (g), volume in litres (l), amount of substance in moles (mol) and molar concentrations (M). The metric system uses multiples of 10 to express decimals. The table below gives the multiplication factor, prefix and symbol for the full range. Chemicals used for biological and physiological research are usually at very low concentrations in the lower milli (m) and micro (μ) areas. However you should also be familiar with the other terms. You may find it useful to practise converting from an exponential multiplication factor to a prefix and symbol, as both ways of expressing concentration are routinely used.

Table 3.1 Metric system multiples

Factor	Prefix	Symbol
10^{-15}	femto	f
10^{-12}	pico	p
10^{-9}	nano	n
10^{-6}	micro	μ
10^{-3}	milli	m
10^{-2}	centi	c
10^{-1}	deci	d
10	deca	da
10^{2}	hecto	h
10^{3}	kilo	k
10^{6}	mega	M
10^{9}	giga	G
10^{12}	tera	T
10^{15}	peta	P

Example 3.1

Q: What would 1457 µg be when expressed in g?

A: µg is 10^{-6} so 1457×10^{-6} g is exactly the same

Example 3.2

Q: What volume would 0.032 l be when expressed as ml?

A: ml is 10^{-3} so you need to move the decimal place 3 places to the right = **32.0 ml**

Example 3.3

Q: How could you express 7.39×10^{-8} M using a prefix instead of a factor?

A: nM is 10^{-9}, which is the nearest prefix, so 73.9×10^{-9} becomes **73.9 nM**

Using grams, litres and volumes

A helpful concept that you will find useful to consider, before making up solutions, is the relationship between the mass of a solution and the volume that solution then takes up. For pure water the definition of volume was dictated by an absolute mass; in other words, one kilogram of water is by definition exactly a litre. The absolute definition has moved on a little now,[1,2,3] but for all practical purposes we can assume that this is still true. You can therefore use this information to 'guestimate' how much volume a certain mass of reagent may take up when made up in solution. This is helpful for choosing the right size container to make up that solution in, and also for developing your sense of what is 'right'. If you know roughly what 100 µl of water looks like in a microcentrifuge tube, then you should be able to spot by eye an inaccurate pipette that has only given you 60 µl.

If you have an accurate enough balance you can use the concept that 100 µl of water should weigh exactly 100 mg to check the accuracy and precision of the pipettes you are using. This is something that will probably be routinely done in your lab, possibly by the technical support staff, or maybe by an outside specialist. However it can be useful to know how to check whether the pipetting errors you are perhaps seeing are due to a badly calibrated pipette, or your bad technique! The simple way to check this is to pipette the same volume of distilled water into a container on a balance four or five times, noting the mass each time. If you continually come up with, for instance, 96 mg, then you would know that your technique is consistent, but that the pipette is consistently calibrated low. This would be a precise, but not accurate pipette! If you get a range of values, e.g. from 95 mg to 107 mg, then you would need to look very carefully at the way you were using the pipette, and/or if it was damaged in some way, as this would indicate a pipette which was accurate(ish) but not precise. You may identify in your lab the set that are usually reliable, and those whose calibration always seems a little off. You may also identify that you need to get some practice in accurate, precise pipetting! Obviously if you want your experiments to be successful, and to give you reliable data, then you need to make sure you use only the reliable set of pipettes, and that you use them correctly! For more information on pipette accuracy and precision, check the literature/manuals that arrived with your pipettes, or the manufacturer's website.[4]

Molarity

The molecular weight of a substance is the addition of the atomic masses of all of its component atoms. For example, glucose has an atomic mass of 180 amu (atomic mass units) i.e. 12 hydrogen atoms with amu of 1, 6 carbon atoms with an amu of 12, 6 oxygen atoms with an amu of 16. Thus $(12 \times 1) + (6 \times 12) + (6 \times 16)$ gives you a total of 180. Often this will be referred to as the relative formula mass (RFM), formula weight (FW) or molecular weight (MW). This information will always be displayed on the label of any compound (*see* Figure 3.1).

One mole of any substance contains by definition 6.023×10^{23} molecules (Avagadro's number). Now 180 g of glucose is the gram molecular weight, and is called a mole. We can calculate how many moles of a substance we have using the weight in grams and the molecular weight according to the equation:

number of moles = mass in grams/molecular weight
moles = mass (g)/MW

This is a very important and useful equation, and conversions from moles to mass to moles is something that you may need to do on a daily basis.

Example 3.4

Q: How many moles are there in 25 g of NaCl? (MW of NaCl is 58.44)

A: moles = 25/58.44 = **0.428 moles**

Obviously if you had 58.44 g of NaCl, then you would have 1 mole.

More usually you will be told that you need to make up a reagent to give a certain number of moles, e.g. 0.5 moles, and so will need to calculate how much to weigh out by rearranging the equation.

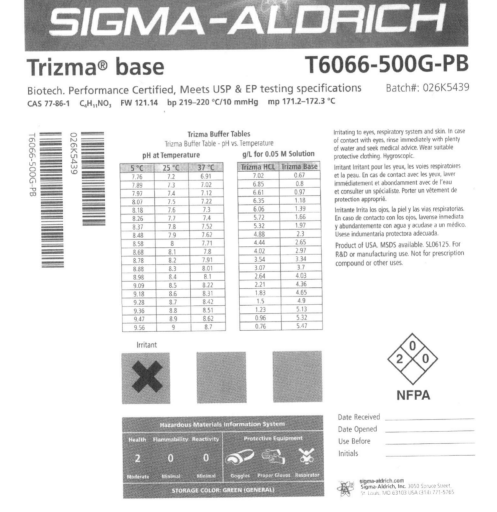

SIGMA-ALDRICH

Trizma® base   T6066-500G-PB

Biotech. Performance Certified, Meets USP & EP testing specifications   Batch#: 026K5439

CAS 77-86-1 $C_4H_{11}NO_3$ FW 121.14   bp 219–220 °C/10 mmHg   mp 171.2–172.3 °C

Trizma Buffer Tables
Trizma Buffer Table - pH vs. Temperature

pH at Temperature			g/L for 0.05 M Solution	
5 °C	25 °C	37 °C	Trizma HCL	Trizma Base
7.76	7.2	6.91	7.02	0.67
7.89	7.3	7.02	6.85	0.8
7.97	7.4	7.12	6.61	0.97
8.07	7.5	7.22	6.35	1.18
8.18	7.6	7.3	6.06	1.39
8.26	7.7	7.4	5.72	1.66
8.37	7.8	7.52	5.32	1.97
8.48	7.9	7.62	4.88	2.3
8.58	8	7.71	4.44	2.65
8.68	8.1	7.8	4.02	2.97
8.78	8.2	7.91	3.54	3.34
8.88	8.3	8.01	3.07	3.7
8.98	8.4	8.1	2.64	4.03
9.09	8.5	8.22	2.21	4.36
9.18	8.6	8.31	1.83	4.65
9.28	8.7	8.42	1.5	4.9
9.36	8.8	8.51	1.23	5.13
9.47	8.9	8.62	0.96	5.32
9.56	9	8.7	0.76	5.47

Irritating to eyes, respiratory system and skin. In case of contact with eyes, rinse immediately with plenty of water and seek medical advice. Wear suitable protective clothing. Hygroscopic.

Irritant Irritant pour les yeux, les voies respiratoires et la peau. En cas de contact avec les yeux, laver immédiatement et abondamment avec de l'eau et consulter un spécialiste. Porter un vêtement de protection approprié.

Irritante Irrita los ojos, la piel y las vias respiratorias. En caso de contacto con los ojos, lavense inmediata y abundante con agua y acudase a un médico. Usese indumentaria protectora adecuada.

Product of USA. MSDS available. SL06125. For R&D or manufacturing use. Not for prescription compound or other uses.

Irritant

NFPA

Health	Flammability	Reactivity
2	0	0

Hazardous Materials Information System

Health	Flammability	Reactivity	Protective Equipment
2	0	0	Goggles Proper Gloves Respirator
Moderate	Minimal	Minimal	

STORAGE COLOR: GREEN (GENERAL)

Date Received _____
Date Opened _____
Use Before _____
Initials _____

sigma-aldrich.com
Sigma-Aldrich, Inc. 3050 Spruce Street,
St. Louis, MO 63103 USA (314) 771-5765

Figure 3.1 Example of a chemical compound label. This label from a chemical compound tub is packed with useful information about the contents, of which the formula weight (FW; also called relative formula mass (RFM) or formula mass (FM)) is essential for calculations to work out how much chemical is needed to make up a particular concentration of reagent. Image courtesy of Sigma-Aldrich Corporation.

Example 3.5

Q: How much would you need to weigh out to have 0.2 moles of NaCl?

A: moles $\times$ MW = mass (g)

0.2 $\times$ 58.44 = 11.69 g

For most biological experiments you will need to use chemicals to make up reagents such as buffers, as per the protocol, which will specify what concentration these should be at.

If you weighed out 180 g of glucose and dissolved it into 1 litre of water, you would have produced a solution with a molarity of 1. This is the definition of a 1 molar solution. Thus molecular weight, concentration and volume are related according to this equation, which we can use to make a molar solution:

moles = concentration (molar) $\times$ volume (l)

Example 3.6

Q: How many moles are there in 2 l of a 0.5 M solution of glucose?

A: moles = 0.5 $\times$ 2 = 1 mole

To calculate the concentration of a solution containing a certain number of moles in a certain volume, you need to rearrange the equation, as shown here.

Example 3.7

Q: If you have 0.1 moles of Na_2HPO_4 in 500 ml, what is the concentration?

A: moles/volume (l) = concentration (M)

= 0.1/0.5

= **0.2 M**

So if you are asked to make up 200 ml of a 0.1 M solution of NaCl (MW 58.44), you can use both equations to help you work out how much to weigh out:

> ### Example 3.8
>
> moles = concentration × volume
> moles = 0.1 × 0.2 = 0.02 moles
> moles × RFM = mass
> 0.02 × 58.44 = 1.17g

So 1.17 g of NaCl added to 200 ml of water will give you a solution with a molar concentration of 0.1 M. Just what you wanted!

Final concentrations

You may be asked to write a working protocol for a technique from a published paper, part of a thesis or a previous student's report or lab book. These will probably describe solutions and reagents as *final concentrations*. A final concentration tells you the molar concentration of a particular reagent in the final total volume of the reaction solution, and not the concentration that the reagent was made up at. Thus to repeat the reaction you will have to work backwards and calculate what concentration you will need to make up, and what volume you will need to achieve the same final concentration. Though at first glance it may seem unnecessarily lengthy, this system is used so that other workers can more easily adapt a method to their own needs, scaling up or down the volumes or numbers as required. You will be expected to write papers and present any reports in this way too. This means that even if you are given a protocol with simple 'add A to B' recipes already calculated, you would still need to calculate the final concentrations you are working at.

> ### Example 3.9
>
> . . . the test sample (50 µl) was incubated with 0.2 mM of reagent A in pH 7.0 phosphate buffer in a total volume of 1 ml and . . .
>
> If reagent A has an RFM of 289.2, how would you make up a solution to do this reaction for 10 samples?

One way to do this would be to make a 10× stock solution of reagent A (2 mM), then add 100 µl of this to the 50 µl test sample and make up to

1000 μl with the phosphate buffer which dilutes reagent A by 10× to give you a final concentration of 0.2 mM. Thus for 10 samples you would perhaps think that you would need to make up 10×100 μl = 1000 μl. However if you only made a total volume of 1000 μl, you would find it very difficult to extract 10 lots of 100 μl. A good tip is to always make up some extra to allow for wastage within the tube. Therefore making up 1200 μl would be a more practical approach.

So we now know that we want 1200 μl of 2 mM reagent A. All we need to do now is calculate how much of reagent A to weigh out using the equations previously described:

Example 3.9 *continued*

$$\begin{aligned}
\text{moles} &= 2 \text{ mM} \times 1200 \text{ μl} \\
&= 2 \times 10^{-3} \text{ M} \times 1200 \times 10^{-6} \text{ l} \\
&= 2.4 \times 10^{-6} \text{ moles}
\end{aligned}$$
$$\begin{aligned}
\text{mass of A} &= 2.4 \times 10^{-6} \times 289.2 \\
&= 694.08 \times 10^{-6} \text{ g} \\
&= \mathbf{0.694 \text{ mg}} \\
&= \mathbf{694 \text{ μg}}
\end{aligned}$$

So adding 694 μg of reagent A to 1200 μl would give you a stock solution of 2 mM, which, when 100 μl was added to the sample and buffer, would result in a final concentration of 0.2 mM, and you have enough to do it 10 times.

This is not the only way to do this but you must always consider what is practical. Weighing out extremely small amounts of a substance is very difficult. Often a better approach is to make up a more concentrated solution and dilute it appropriately, when you need to use it. These are sometimes referred to as *stock solutions*. You may also need to consider the cost of the reagent, whether you have lots or only a little to use, whether other people are going to use it too. Care must also be taken when moving between mM, μM, ml and μl. You may find it easier to put everything into M, g and l and use exponential notation (as above) to avoid losing a factor of 10 or even 1000!

pH

The term pH refers to the concentration of free hydrogen ions $[H^+]$ in a solution. They are related via this equation:

$$pH = \log_{10} 1/[H^+] = -\log_{10} [H^+]$$

The measurable range extends from pH 1, very acidic, with a high free $[H^+]$ concentration of 0.1 M, to pH 14, very alkali, with a $[H^+]$ of 1×10^{-14} M. However biological systems generally only tolerate a narrow range near to neutral pH 7 and are very, very sensitive to changes in pH. This means that a badly made buffer which is too acid or too alkali may prevent the expected reaction or biological interaction from proceeding in the correct manner.[5]

Thus you must always take care when preparing solutions to ensure that they are made up to the appropriate pH. This may involve correcting the pH by adding an acid or alkali to adjust the $[H^+]$. pH of solutions is usually measured using a pH meter, which has an electrode that can measure the electrical potential of a solution and display it in standard pH units. Operating instructions vary from machine to machine, but generally they are calibrated using standard solutions of *known* pH. You should always make sure the meter is correctly calibrated before you begin to use it, that your solution is being properly stirred when measuring and correcting the pH, but that the electrode (which is very fragile and expensive to replace) is not in danger of being damaged by the stirrer. Correction is usually done with 1 M HCl to make things more acidic or 1 M NaOH to make things more alkali. Sometimes these reagents are not appropriate (for certain buffers), so always check what is required for the solution you are making.

Example 3.10

Q: You need to make up a buffer with a pH of 6.5; the pH meter reading says that the pH after adding all of the reagents is 8.7. What do you need to add?

A: The pH of the solution is currently too alkali, therefore to make it more acidic, add 1 M HCl dropwise.

Dilutions

Reagents are often prepared as a concentrated stock that has to be diluted before use. Sometimes a reagent is required at a whole range of different concentrations or dilutions. Molar solutions are not the only way to express this; sometimes percentage solutions are also used.

Example 3.11

Q: How would you prepare 1 l of a 5% (w/v) solution of sucrose?

A: w/v stands for weight/volume, so 5% is 5 g weight in a 100 ml volume. To make up 1 l multiply by 10
   = 50 g sucrose in 1000 ml

Similarly percentage solutions can be used when diluting a liquid reagent, (v/v) or volume/volume solutions.

Example 3.12

Q: How would you make up 500 ml of a 20% (v/v) solution of methanol?

A: 20% = 20 ml methanol in 100 ml, i.e. add 20 ml to 80 ml to reach 100 ml final volume. For 500 ml multiply by 5.
   = 100 ml methanol added to 400 ml water

For molar solutions you can calculate how to dilute your stock reagent to give you the right concentration (conc) in the right volume (vol) by using this equation:

(final conc wanted/initial conc) × final vol wanted (ml)
= vol of initial conc (ml) needed

Example 3.13

Q: You have reagent X at a stock concentration of 0.5 mM and you need to prepare 100 ml of 0.01 mM working solution. How would you do it?

A: (final conc/initial conc) × final volume = (0.01/0.5) × 100 = **2 ml**

So 2 ml of 0.5 mM stock added to 98 ml water gives you 100 ml of 0.01 mM working solution.

A range of concentrations of a reagent can be prepared via serial dilutions. This method involves making up a starting stock solution at the highest concentration needed, and then serially diluting some of the stock to cover a range. This is much more accurate than making up multiple solutions from scratch. The calculations can be difficult, as you use some of the previous dilution to make up the next, but you also need to ensure that you make up enough volume of each concentration to use in the actual experiment! Again a good tip is to err on the side of caution and always make up a little extra.

Example 3.14

Q: You need to make up protein Z for a dose–response experiment at a range of concentrations from 1 M to 1×10^{-6} M, diluting by $10\times$ each time. At least 1 ml of each concentration is required. How will you do it?

This is a 10-fold dilution at each step 1 M, 0.1 M, 0.01 M down to 0.000001 M or 1×10^{-6} M, and so this is a fairly straightforward serial dilution. The minimum volume is 1 ml, so making up 1.5 ml (or 1500 µl) will ensure that we have more than enough.

A: Using the equation:
  $(0.1/1.0) \times 1500$ µl $= 150$ µl
  So 150 µl of 1 M solution + 1350 µl $H_2O \rightarrow 1500$ µl of 0.1 M solution

This is enough to use for the experiment (1 ml) and leaves 500 µl to make the next dilution. This is also a 10-fold dilution so the answer is the same:

$(0.01/0.1) \times 1500$ µl $= 150$ µl

So:

150 µl of 0.1 M solution + 1350 µl $H_2O \rightarrow 1500$ µl of 0.01 M solution

So now we have three of our solutions, and just need to carry on making dilutions in the same way until we reach 1×10^{-6} M. This final solution will have a volume of 1500 µl, but because we do not need to make a further dilution, there will be excess, which we do not use.

150 µl of 0.1 M solution + 1350 µl $H_2O \rightarrow 1500$ µl of 0.01 M solution
150 µl of 0.01 M solution + 1350 µl $H_2O \rightarrow 1500$ µl of 0.001 M solution
150 µl of 1×10^{-3} M solution + 1350 µl $H_2O \rightarrow 1500$ µl of 1×10^{-4} M solution
150 µl of 1×10^{-4} M solution + 1350 µl $H_2O \rightarrow 1500$ µl of 1×10^{-5} M solution
150 µl of 1×10^{-5} M solution + 1350 µl $H_2O \rightarrow 1500$ µl of 1×10^{-6} M solution

This serial dilution covers a wide range from 1 M down to 1×10^{-6} M. Sometimes the dilution factors are much less.

Example 3.15

Q: You need to make up a 50 μl sample of protein Q for a standard curve. The range is from 10 mM to 2 mM in steps of 2 mM.

If we decide to make up 150 μl to have extra, the first dilution would look like this:

A: $(8/10) \times 150$ μl = 120 μl
   120 μl of 10 mM solution + 30 μl $H_2O \rightarrow$ 150 μl of 8 mM solution

This seems OK, but if we calculate the next step we can see there is a problem:

$(6/8) \times 150$ μl = 112.5 μl
112.5 μl of 8 mM solution + 37.5 μl $H_2O \rightarrow$ 150 μl of 6 mM solution

We need to use 112.5 μl of the 0.8 mM dilution to make up the next dilution, but as we only made 150 μl, this would only leave 37.5 μl for the experiment, not the 50 μl minimum that we need.
   Thus with a dilution where the factor is less than 2-fold, more of the concentrated solution than water goes into the next dilution, and so you will need to make up a higher volume of each of the earlier dilutions in order to have enough to make the full range. Often it can be helpful to work backwards, and calculate how much of the *last* concentration you need (with a little excess). You can then decide how much of the previous dilution will be needed, plus the volume needed for the experiment. This is quite a difficult serial dilution, so don't worry if it seems confusing at first. You just need to keep juggling the numbers until you have a sensible plan! Here we start with the most dilute, 2 mM:

$(2/4) \times 100$ μl = 50 μl
∴ 50 μl of 4 mM solution + 50 μl $H_2O \rightarrow$ 100 μl of 2 mM solution
$(4/6) \times 150$ μl = 100 μl
∴ 100 μl of 6 mM solution + 50 μl $H_2O \rightarrow$ 150 μl of 4 mM solution, 50 μl for the experiment, 100 μl left
$(6/8) \times 200$ μl = 150 μl
∴ 150 μl of 8 mM solution + 50 μl $H_2O \rightarrow$ 200 μl of 6 mM solution, 50 μl for the experiment, 150 μl left
$(8/10) \times 250$ μl = 200 μl

$\therefore$ 200 µl of 10 mM solution + 50 µl $H_2O \rightarrow$ 250 µl of 8 mM solution, 50 µl for the experiment, 200 µl left

There is still a margin of excess of about 50 µl, and so there is enough to make all of the dilutions and do the experiments.

With all the calculations discussed in this section it is important that you do all the work in your lab book before you go near the lab and start setting up tubes! If you are not sure you have it right (or even if you are), it is always a good idea to get it checked by someone else, e.g. a graduate student, post doc or even your supervisor. It is much better to get a new calculation checked out and confirmed before you dive in and use up the last 10 g of an expensive reagent that takes 6 weeks to be shipped in from the US when you really only needed 10 µg!

References

1   National Institute of Standards and Technology. *Reference on Constants, Units and Uncertainty*. http://physics.nist.gov/cuu/Units/ (accessed 25 June 2006).
2   Rowlett R and The University of North Carolina at Chapel Hill. *How Many? A Dictionary of Units of Measurement*. www.unc.edu/~rowlett/units/dictK.html (accessed 25 June 2006).
3   Tapson F. *A Dictionary of Units*. Exeter: University of Exeter. www.ex.ac.uk/cimt/dictunit/dictunit.htm#volume (accessed 25 June 2006).
4   Anachem Lifetime Pipette Care. www.anachem.co.uk/anachem/lifescience/page. asp?Pagename=Inaccuracy/Imprecision (accessed 25 June 2006).
5   Morris JG. *A Biologist's Physical Chemistry* (2e). London: Edward Arnold; 1974.

Chapter 4

Designing and managing experiments

Planning

The key to successful research and productive experimentation is complete and effective planning. No-one can (or should) walk into a lab and dive straight in! This may seem a little dull if you are raring to get going, but good planning will always save you time and give you better results in the long run! Time spent deciding *what* to do, *how* to do it and *when* to do it is an essential part of your research (possibly the most important part . . .), and is a skill that you must work to develop.

At the beginning of the project your supervisor will probably have everything mapped out for you, but this will only be for the first few weeks or so; they do not have time (or the inclination) to plan every day for you for the duration of your project. Once you start to get to grips with the techniques and procedures, you should start to take over your own experimental designs.

There is more than one way of organising your experiments, and you may have try out a few different methods in order to find the one that suits your working style and the type of research you are involved in. For any hypothesis-driven experimentation there are a few general guidelines that you can use to help your planning:

- make sure you know what you are trying to show: have a clear hypothesis or inquiry that you want your experiments to answer
- take time to make sure that the experiment you have planned will actually address the question(s) you have asked
- decide if the method you have chosen is the most appropriate way of proceeding – is there an easier/cheaper/quicker/cleverer way?
- have a rough idea what kind of results you might get: be already thinking, 'if I get x then it means y, but if I get z it means a, b and c'
- be thinking ahead to any potential problems with the plan, e.g. technical failures, false results etc, and plan how you will deal with them
- be prepared to change your hypotheses when the results come in – be open-minded and flexible enough to amend your ideas (even your pet

theories) in the light of new data. This is how all research moves forward!

- make sure you have the correct skills/information to perform the experiments correctly and safely. If not, you may need to undertake some training; this may be a formal course or a quick 15 minute tutorial by another member of the team
- experiments often just don't work; be systematic, analytical, dogged and determined and you *will* make progress.

In an ideal world the only considerations you would have to take into account would be what you needed for your work. However in the real world, in a practical working lab there are many other things that have an impact on how you design your experiments!

Time management is the first issue and will be discussed fully later on in this chapter, but experimental planning always has to take timescales into consideration. For instance, if your protocol takes three days to complete, don't start it on a Thursday unless you want to spend Saturday in the lab. If you do, fine, but if you have to have a more senior member of staff to supervise you, you'd better make sure they want to spend their weekend with you too!

For experiments using cultured cells (which take time to grow, and need to be fed regularly), experiments involving animals or animal tissues, equipment with a high usage etc, forward planning is extremely important. Many shared items of specialised or expensive pieces of equipment such as microscopes, cryostats, spectrophotometers, sequencers etc often have a booking system – a diary where you book hours of time for your own use. If a system like this is in use, then do not make a booking unless you are sure you are going to need to use the equipment. Be aware that other people need to use it too; do not block-book days at a time, only book what you really are going to use. If you find you cannot use your slot then let people know so someone else can make use of the extra time. This kind of common courtesy can mean a great deal in a busy lab, and will make the other researchers much more likely to help you when you get stuck.

If you have a lot of samples to analyse or test then you may need a long-term planner to be able to organise your experiments. An experiment that runs overnight may mean you can only run it four or five times in a standard working week; thus in order to estimate when you should have preliminary data, booking up your own time for that experiment for months to come can often be the best way. You can also see how much of each reagent you will need and when it will need to be reordered; and can build in other experiments or tasks around it. This concept of making the most productive use of your time leads us into the realm of 'time management'.

Time management

Your time in the lab is precious, and in order for you to get the best possible results you need to use it wisely. This means that along with careful planning of your experiments, you must plan in time for other things such as reading and keeping up to date with the literature, analysing your data, preparing for lab meetings and writing for eventual publications. There is more than one method of managing your time, but it must fit with your experimental planning so you always have a firm grip on your activities. If the pressure is on to produce good results, then it becomes more important than ever that your finite time is as productive as possible.[1]

It doesn't matter whether you use a diary, wall chart or a personal digital assistant (PDA); you should have a clear system for planning, logging and tracking your activities, both in the lab and out. Here you can plot those long-term experimental sets, and decide how to fit in your other tasks around them. It can be used to build in preparation time for future objectives as well as enabling you to focus clearly on the correct aspect of the task in hand. Using a diary in this way takes discipline, and a half-hearted effort is likely to be counterproductive.

Take time to prioritise your tasks – don't allow yourself to spend too much time doing easy or fun jobs at the expense of important but dull jobs. Breaking large jobs into many smaller ones can make them less daunting, and is a useful strategy when you come to write up your projects and produce papers. Lists can be a useful way of keeping track of where you are and what you need to do (if you are a list person . . .). This can be very important when doing a series of similar (or the same) experiment on many hundreds of samples, or when working through a range of different tests on the same sample.

Box 4.1   Top tips for time management

- Set aside some time each day to review your tasks for that day: prioritise tasks and assign timescales. This may build into weekly/monthly planning meetings with your supervisor or team leader.
- Make sure the goals you are working towards are really what you *and* your supervisor wants. Don't be distracted into 'interesting'

sidelines that use up your time and result in the main job taking longer.

- Manage your workspace; keep your desk area and lab areas clean and tidy. Efficient organisation means that you won't waste time hunting for that important paper, or the latest data that you want to plot. Keep on top of filing papers or results etc, so that it never becomes a big job. This of course has health and safety implications too.

- Use slow lab time such as incubations to work on other tasks such as preparing the reagents for the next stage, or catching up on the literature. Some tasks are flexible (such as reading), others must be done at a certain time for the experiment to succeed. Identify these 'immovable tasks' and organise everything else around them. This 'jigsaw' approach helps you to stay on top of the smaller tasks without affecting the long-term planning of your major experiments.

Controls

Without controls your results can mean absolutely nothing. Controls prove that you have done what you think you've done, and that the results that you get are a product of that experiment and they aren't just due to chance or a mistake. Appropriate, correctly used controls make your data more robust and more likely to be taken seriously; marks are often lost from good project reports, and papers are turned down by journals because of the apparent lack of adequate controls. This is easily avoided, but needs serious consideration. Do not be fooled into thinking that controls are something that you just tag on the end of an experiment. Controls are central to any experiment and are an essential tool for diagnosing any problems that arise within the experiment. They should be built into the experimental plan from the very beginning and, in a way, can be the most important part. Certainly 'bad' controls can devalue or even negate even the most illuminating and exciting experimental data.

Controls can be broadly split into two groups – positive and negative. Negative controls are experiments that are missing a fundamental reagent or sample and should not work. These are often called 'blanks'. Sometimes they may consist solely of water or buffer, such as in a polymerase chain reaction (PCR). Any product DNA that is found in this control shows that there has been contamination and that all of the other products should be viewed with suspicion. Other types of negative control may contain all of the reagents for a reaction *except* the sample to be tested, and therefore give a measure of the background activity of the reagents. This value is then deducted from the sample results. Controls like these can be especially useful if there is a problem with degradation of one of the reagents into something else, which might give a false positive. If a toxin or inhibitor effect were being measured, the control would contain no toxin/inhibitor, to show the normal level of activity of the effect being studied. Generally any 'positive' measurement gained from a negative control should ring alarm bells and should start you on a hunt to identify the problem.

Positive controls are a set-up in which you include something you know will definitely give you a good result. For example, in an assay testing enzyme levels in tissue extracts, a good positive control would be pure enzyme brought in from a chemical supplier and used in excess. This will always give a high reading and shows that all of the reagents are working correctly. If the positive control fails to give a result, then you know that there is a problem with the reagents. If your samples show nothing but the positive is good, then you can be more confident in saying that you have no (or very little) enzyme present (*see* Table 4.1 for an example).

Often you will need multiple controls, both positive and negative, to check that both the 'test' you are using is working correctly and that the 'experiment' is working correctly. For example, in a western blot (*see* Chapter 7) you could run one lane with the extract from a cell line *known* to express your protein of interest as a positive control for the technique, and one lane with an extract from a cell line known *not* to express your protein. Thus your positive should always come up, and your negative should not. Any variation in this outcome means that you may have a problem, perhaps a cross-reaction of the primary antibody, and whatever your test sample tells you, you know that there is a fault with the method and that you cannot use the results without further investigation.

Table 4.1 Example of positive and negative control data

Sample type	Reading (units)	Comments
Negative control	15	Low, showing background activity
Positive control	896	High, showing all reagents are working
Sample 1	159	Measurable samples
Sample 2	269	Measurable samples
Sample 3	377	Measurable samples
Sample 4	18	Very little activity – repeat?

Duplication and repetition

An experiment that gives you a particular result only once is not reliable, and you cannot believe the data that it produces. If you get roughly the same answer more than once but there are wide variations, then your results are not accurate. These kinds of results may be useful for planning further, more refined experiments, or for gaining new insights and prompting ideas (*'fishing expeditions'*), but they are not publishable. In order for you to publish your data in any way it must be reproducible and accurate. This means that for any given experiment when you repeat it under the same conditions, you should get the same answer within acceptable limits. How can you achieve this type of 'robust' data?

Good experimental planning and repetition improves accuracy and reliability. Wherever possible do your experiments as duplicates, or, better still, triplicates. The mean of the results will be more accurate, and by looking at the spread between the samples you can see how reproducible your experiment is. When using animals, precious human samples or expensive reagents this can be difficult but should always be included wherever possible. An amazingly interesting result is useless unless it can be repeated and be shown to be true on more than one occasion, in samples taken from different animals/cultures etc. Bear this in mind when planning your experimental timetable – don't put all of your eggs into one basket and do all of one set together in one afternoon. You may have a bad set of reagents, or an accidental spillage. Splitting experimental groups over different days and test runs again can bolster your data if your results remain consistent. This can also be a useful tool for spotting external effects that may be affecting your work. If you only get that surprising spike on your patch-clamp readout on mornings when the builders are drilling, you may have to re-evaluate the possible causes!

When an experiment is repeated and the data produced are similar but not exactly the same you need to decide if they fall within an acceptable spread, i.e. you are happy with the errors. There are various ways you can estimate errors for an experiment, the simplest being to look at all of the measurements you make over the whole technique and make reasonable predictions about the number of significant figures or plus/minus ranges to take readings to. For example if you can count cells to an accuracy of only to the nearest hundred, then two results within 500 of each other would be acceptable as being the 'same'. Two results 5000 cells different would sit less happily in a single treatment group!

Increasing the 'n' number can also help with the accuracy; for many purposes (sets of cells, animals etc) $n = 4$ is the minimum you can use if you hope to do any kind of statistical analysis, and $n = 6$ would always be better! While this book does not address the use of statistics in science (that would be a whole book by itself . . .), it can be helpful to consider what kind of analysis may be made at the end of the experiment when thinking about setting up the test groups at the beginning of the experiment! Some tests require a much larger n of 20 or more; data that are only semi-quantitative may not be analysable in this way at all, and so other techniques will need to be used to ensure reliability.

Keeping careful track of the reagents used in each experiment can also be helpful for improving the robustness of experiments, and becomes invaluable if any problems arise. Often a set of less reliable results or failed experiments can be tracked to a badly made buffer or batch of contaminated media. Thus you should get into the habit not only of labelling clearly all of your reagents with your name, the contents and production dates, but you should be tying this information to the sets of experiments the reagents were used for, and to the stock sources the reagents were made from (*see* Table 4.2 for an example). This produces a 'paper trail' you can follow if (and when) problems arise. This is especially important if there is a delay between setting or performing experiments and the data being produced. Sometimes weeks or months may have elapsed, which would make it very difficult to remember exactly which batch was at fault.

If you have an unusual/surprising/interesting result, that you can reproduce using different sets of reagents made from different stock supplies, for multiple sets of samples/animals/cells, then you can be confident that you have a real result. Often the first thing that you will be challenged on with any result you produce will be the conditions under which you have produced that result. Start as you mean to go on, by planning the 'robustness' into your experiments, and you can always be confident that your technique is sound, and therefore your data are accurate and reliable.

Table 4.2 Example of a paper trail tracking stock and working reagents

Experiment number	Buffer A made	From stock made
2: OK	10 May 2005	9 May 2005
3: OK	11 May 2005	9 May 2005
4: bad data	13 May 2005	13 May 2005, query stock OK?
5: bad data	17 May 2005	13 May 2005
6: OK	20 May 2005	19 May 2005

Reagents and ordering

Most labs carry a limited stock of the most commonly used reagents. All will have the basics, such as NaCl, for buffers, plus the rare chemicals needed only for the specific work that lab is doing. Other supplies include assay kits, antibodies, DNA samples, cell cultures, tissue banks etc. You may find yourself surprised at the costs of some things; assay kits can cost upwards of £300, and rare cell types are effectively priceless. Make sure you are aware of these precious resources and treat them accordingly. Pay attention to the stock levels of the items you are using, and let someone know if they are running low, so that orders can be placed in good time. Bear in mind that other people may need to use the same chemicals as you! Some items can be ordered and will arrive the next day if in stock (Sigma), others come from further afield, or are subject to delay. Don't end up wasting three weeks of your project time waiting for a reagent to arrive, because you didn't tell your supervisor that you needed some more until it was all gone.

Different labs will all have their own order placement system that you would do well to familiarise yourself with. You will also initially need to have any orders you want to place checked and countersigned, usually by your supervisor or lab manager. Again, forward planning is vital if no-one else can sign and your supervisor is going to be away for two weeks!

Reference

1   Hindle T. *Manage Your Time*. London: Dorling Kindersley; 1998.

Chapter 5

Keeping track of data

Graphs

Graphs are an excellent way of presenting numerical information in a pictorial manner. Good graphs promote understanding of the results by simplifying lots of data into a single image. They should help the reader to interpret the meaning and relationships between the sets of information being compared. Bad graphs are confusing, vague, misleading and sometimes downright fraudulent!

There are many kinds of graphs, but all should have the same fundamental elements. Failure to include all of these things renders a graph useless and can mean a report or paper being misunderstood or rejected for publication. Box 5.1 is a checklist that you can use to make sure that all of your graphs have the basics in place.

Box 5.1 Basic 'musts' for good graphs

- *Title*: this may include an identifying number/code.
- *Labels on both axes*: make sure that you include the correct units where appropriate.
- *An appropriate scale*: always start at 0 if possible (unless you need negative numbers) and only go up to a round value just above the highest point.
- *Legend*: clearly identifying the different sets of data where appropriate.
- *Include error bars* and make it clear if they are standard error or standard deviation.
- *Choose statistical markers carefully* and clearly include the *P* value or test that they refer to.
- *Use a figure legend*: this can help explain what the graph is trying to show.

You need to consider some additional factors to make sure your graphs have the maximum positive impact (*see* Box 5.2).

Box 5.2 Giving your data the right impact

- *Choose the right kind of graph*: line graphs for continuous data, bar or column for discrete data. These are probably all you will need for a scientific report.
- *Don't put too much data on one graph*: it just gets muddled and confusing.
- *Don't be tempted by 3D effects or other flashy styles*: keep things clear and simple.
- *Don't use shaded backgrounds or gridlines*: these are default on some software packages and so will need to be removed.
- *Use the correct font size for the text*, not too big or too small.
- *Be careful with your use of colours*: keep the axis and text black and stick to a simple colour scheme for the markers/lines/columns.
- If you are presenting the same type of data on many graphs, try and stick with a consistent colour scheme, e.g. control samples always in green, treated samples in red.
- If two or more graphs are to be directly compared, draw them side-by-side and use the same scale.
- Do not use stretched or squashed scales to distort the data, however tempting it might be to give you the shape that you want!
- Remember the limitations of your data and don't try to over-extrapolate or force points onto a curve.
- Do not delete data just because you think they don't fit very well; always have a valid scientific reason for including or excluding any data.
- Make it clear what the *n* number is for each data point/bar.

See Figure 5.1 for examples of the way the right and wrong graph can affect how your data are presented. Graphs A and B, C and D, and E and F, have the same data plotted in two different ways to show how bad presentation can distort the way the data looks, and therefore can influence the reader's perception of the results.

In graph A it appears that there is a large difference between the samples, especially 3 and 4 because of the compressed use of the vertical *y* axis scale, while lengthening the axis plot by beginning at 68 instead of 0.

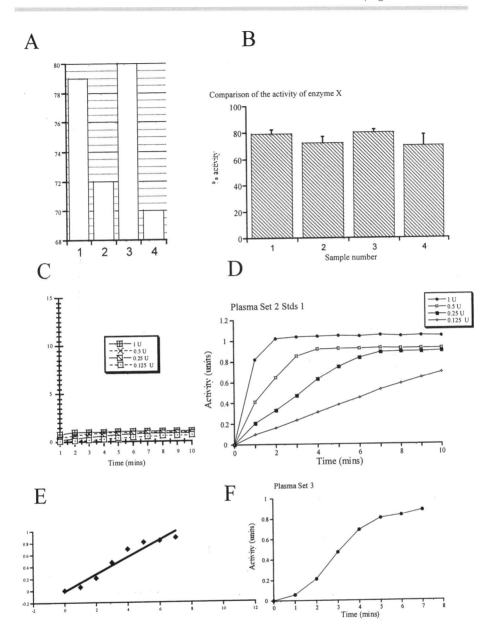

Figure 5.1 Example graphs.

Shortening of the *x* axis and using the (unnecessary) grid also add to the impression of large differences. There are no error bars so we cannot have any idea of the spread or *n* number, which means we do not know how much confidence we should have in the data. We would almost be expecting to see statistical significances here! However if we look at graph B where the y axis begins at 0, and the x axis isn't squashed, we can see that there is no real difference between any of the samples. The clearer graph with simple hatching makes it easier to see what is going on, and the error bars show us that the dataset is quite tight, increasing our confidence in the result. There are no significant differences here!

In graph C the bad scale makes it look as though all of the data are about the same, whereas when the correct scale is used on graph D, the lines are obviously quite different. The unhelpful choice of markers and line hatching in graph C would make it difficult to pick out which line you were looking at even if the scale were better. Graph D uses very simple markers that are not easily confused. If you have access to a colour printer, this type of graph would look better still with coloured markers and lines.

Graph E uses a big thick line of best fit to make the data look as though it is a straight line, when you can see from graph F that it is in fact a rectangular hyperbola. This could totally change the meaning of the data and the subsequent conclusions of the research, and shows how you must take care when using automatic tools in graph-plotting packages. Just because there is a button to curve/line fit your data, doesn't mean you should use it! Always think about what it is you are trying to show, how it fits into your story, and make sure that the data are fairly represented and not crow-barred into the shape that you think they should be in!

Tables

Tables can be used to organise data and present them in a way that highlights trends, describes relationships, and classifies information. As with the graph, simplicity is the key. Tables should be clearly labelled, with column and row headings. These can be emphasised by using bold typescript. During the course of your research you may use tables to collate your data, or to present sections of work to your supervisor. These can be large and complex, but do not be tempted to transfer them straight into written reports or papers. Tables used in publications must be much more concise and only contain information that is essential. It should be easy for the reader to pull out the results they are interested in from the table. Data should never be presented in both a table and a graph. Choose the most appropriate format to say what you want to say and stick to it. *See* Table 5.1 for an example of how a table can be used to organise, collate and manage data; it shows how data can be easily collated and managed in a table. Here the tissue type and treatment, number of samples and data with standard errors of means (sem) are easily accessible, and if the table is

Table **5.1** Example of a data table

Treatment	n	Subtype 1	Subtype 1 sem	Subtype 2	Subtype 2 sem	Total	Total sem
A	6	0.296	0.040	1.471	0.118	1.919	0.150
B	2	0.321	0.017	1.861	0.169	2.391	0.036
C	6	0.303	0.016	1.401	0.053	1.808	0.075
D	2	0.786	0.057	3.169	0.178	4.179	0.229
E	6	0.360	0.014	1.717	0.127	2.296	0.125
F	6	0.262	0.016	1.562	0.053	1.879	0.066
G	6	0.379	0.048	1.093	0.145	1.717	0.216
H	6	0.306	0.019	1.614	0.063	2.116	0.097
I	6	0.496	0.041	1.925	0.067	2.517	0.110
J	6	0.378	0.028	1.240	0.158	1.627	0.105
K	6	0.325	0.016	1.859	0.068	2.347	0.057
L	4	0.463	0.020	1.177	0.102	1.841	0.102

set up before the experiment the data can be added as and when it is produced, helping with the tracking of progress.

Spreadsheets

Spreadsheets can be enormously useful for organising your results. Setting up a standard spreadsheet to perform a repetitive calculation means that you can process your raw data much more efficiently. They can also be used to track your progress through complex experimental set-ups.

It can often be quite time consuming to set up a spreadsheet, but if the calculation/data handling set-up is going to be used a lot over the course of the research then undoubtedly it will be worth it! Depending on your familiarity with spreadsheet software such as MS Excel you can set up sheets for very simple addition, subtraction or summing activities, or for more complex logging of large matrices of detailed information. Using a

Table **5.2** Example of an Excel spreadsheet

	A	B	C	D	E	F	G
1	Sample no.	Raw data	Inc time	vol(ul)	data/min	data/min/ul	Average 1-5
2	1	0.385	10	20	0.0385	0.001925	
3	2	0.412	10	20	0.0412	0.00206	
4	3	0.298	7	20	0.042571	0.002128571	
5	4	0.401	10	20	0.0401	0.002005	
6	5	0.296	7	20	0.042286	0.002114286	**0.002029643**

spreadsheet takes the concept of a data table further than just storage of information by performing simple or complex calculations. In the example shown in Table 5.2, the sheet does basic data handling such as correcting the data to changes per minute and per sample volume, and then finds the average of the sample set automatically.

Spreadsheets can also be a useful way of keeping track of large quantities of data, even if you don't need to perform many calculations. They can be used to feed numerical data into statistical analysis programs or to create graphs or tables for reports and publications. There is (theoretically) no limit to the number of columns/rows you can have, which makes a spreadsheet a powerful tool for organising and handling your data. Don't forget that non-numerical text data and information can also be handled by spreadsheets. As with many computer-based tools, if you don't have the technical skills required to get the most out of the program, it can often be worth your while to embark on a training course. Expertise in using a spreadsheet programme could be the factor that allows you to double the amount of data you can generate and analyse over the course of a research project. Now *that* would make your supervisor happy!

Databases

Databases are another tool for handling quantities of information in an organised manner. As with spreadsheets they can be used for keeping track of both quantitative and non-quantitative information. If you have multiple experimental sets, then setting up a standard 'record' card on which you can log the same type of data every time can be a good way of storing information. Databases (and again there are many kinds) usually allow you to sort the records by different fields and search for keywords or numbers. An example is shown in Figure 5.2; this type of record card can be used to track experimental technical details, which are useful to refer to if ever there is a problem. This example is for a western blotting set-up (*see* Chapter 7) and includes information such as when the gel was poured, and the voltage the gel was run at. If there is a problem later on, this kind of information can, for instance, be used to trace a bad batch of gels.

Databases can also be used to keep track of the literature you have read. Specialised programs such as 'Endnote' can be used to build bibliographies automatically when linked to word processing packages. Often the 'records' can be filled automatically from online library entries, which means you could avoid having to type a single reference for a thesis or paper!

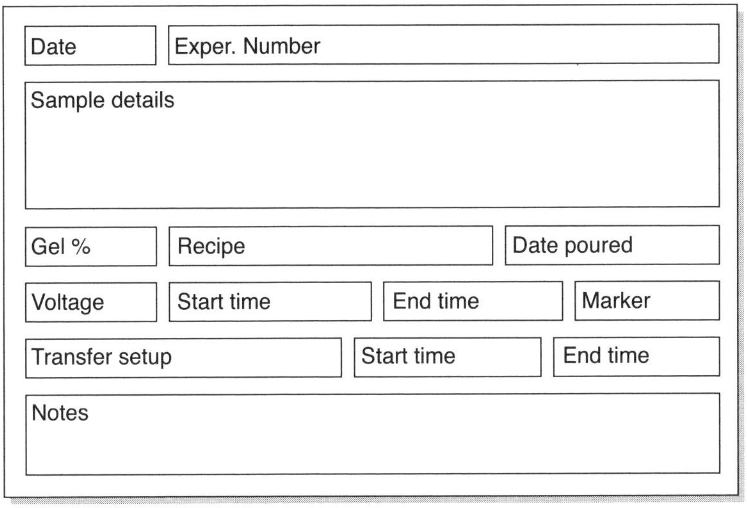

Date	Exper. Number

Sample details

Gel %	Recipe	Date poured

Voltage	Start time	End time	Marker

Transfer setup	Start time	End time

Notes

Figure 5.2 Example of a database record card.

There may be a 'master' list of the core literature for your lab or research group's interests which you could have access to, or perhaps you could begin to build your own . . .

Units

Unit names and prefixes have been covered elsewhere in this handbook (*see* p. 19), so this is just a reminder to take special care to make sure you use the correct units throughout your project, including on the spreadsheets or databases and especially in the final report/paper. Start using the correct units from day one and be consistent. Don't present half of your data one way, and the rest another. This is very confusing and will lead the reader to think that you do not understand what your results are, let alone what they might mean.

Laboratory notebooks

The laboratory notebook is an essential part of your research and should always be maintained in a 'scrutinisable' manner. This book should be a complete record of everything you have done while working on your research project. It should be hardback and bound; a loose-leaf file is generally not acceptable. Every experiment you do should be included in chronological order, clearly dated, and nothing should be omitted. Thus every calculation, weighing for solution preparation, spillage, mistake, etc, etc should be in it. It is also where you can record new ideas, plans for experiments, and current results. Draft graphs, data tables, photos of gels etc can be pasted in. Comments regarding your interpretation of the data should be added as you go along, as you will find these invaluable when you come to write up your results for the report or paper.

Some labs use a double book system where a smaller 'rough' book is taken into the lab, and gets messy; while a 'neat' book (A4) has all of the information from the rough book copied into it each evening. This system is fine as long as the two books are the same and no 'editing' of problems or mistakes is allowed. Check with your supervisor/team leader as to which system they want you to use.

A detailed lab book like this is invaluable when you (inevitably) have problems. An assay that suddenly stops working can often be tracked back through the lab book to a silly mistake in the preparation of a reagent the previous week. This is why you should always write what you actually *did*, not just what you planned to do.

In some labs, and when working for some funding bodies such as those from industry or government departments, the contents of the lab book are a legal document. If your research leads to a new patent or important discovery, then the lab book, written at the time of the experiments, is proof that you did the work, and that you did it correctly. For any controversial or contentious result you may have to use the lab book as evidence of the standard of your work, and to back up your claims. All this means that however scrappy or untidy it may be, your lab book must always be readable and understandable by another researcher. Someone else *must* be able to pick it up and follow exactly what you have been doing; and if necessary repeat it *verbatim* to achieve the same result.

Data sheets

Some experimental results are produced as copious sheets of printed data. This might be absorbance data from a spectrophotometer, radioactive counting data from a scintillation counter, DNA sequences etc, etc. For these data to retain any meaning they must be carefully logged with the experiment number or identifier, date and, if appropriate, the time. They should be kept in an organised fashion, in an A4 folder, wallet file or box file. Again this will be of great help to you when you need to find sections of data to plot graphs and write up your results. The data must be organised so that they can be understood and used by other people.

This idea of administrative transparency keeps on raising its head! Once again, organisation is the key factor to the overall success of your research. The use of spreadsheets and/or databases may again be appropriate.

Catalogue systems

A good habit to get into is to catalogue everything to do with your research project. This means that you assign a number or code to all of your experiments, and this code is then carried through onto the pertinent data sheets, into your lab books, and onto graphs and tables. These codes would not appear in the project report or papers; they are tools for you to use in order to organise and clarify your activities and data. If your project involves the testing of multiple samples, a system of this kind helps you to keep track of your progress and will help you with your experimental planning. An example is shown in Table 5.3.

Table 5.3 Example of an experiment logging system

Experiment number	Date	Samples tested	Data sheet	Lab book page	Comments
RBC1	10 February 2004	27–45	8	4	35 to be repeated
RBC2	12 February 2004	46–70	9–10	6	All OK
PLA1	17 February 2004	2–10, +15	11	9	11–14 not done
PLA2	20 February 2004	11–14, 16–30	12–13	11	All OK

Filing

Keep everything! A small scrap of paper that your supervisor jotted on in the first week may be extremely important and just the thing that you need to sort out that troublesome calculation! Every piece of data, photo, hyperfilm, graph etc should be catalogued and saved – even (perhaps especially) the ones that appear not to have worked. If you have a run of problems, then looking at the last five experiments that gave apparently silly results may help you and your supervisor to pinpoint and solve the problem. Here again, an A4 box file is useful, or you could attach everything to your lab book.

As things become more complicated, an integrated system of lab books, computer spreadsheets, printed graphs etc is essential for you to keep on top of what you are doing with your research and where you are going. If you are working towards a project report or thesis then an organised system like this will make the writing up process go much more smoothly and efficiently. If you had a great result, but you can't put your hand on the data, or find the exact version of the reagent you used to produce it, then your result is meaningless because you cannot justify, defend or repeat it. Be 'scientific' and systematic in your approach, and your research will always benefit.

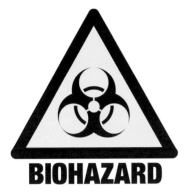
BIOHAZARD

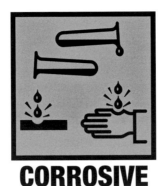
CORROSIVE

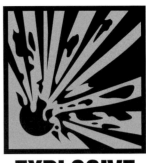
EXPLOSIVE

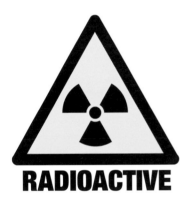
RADIOACTIVE

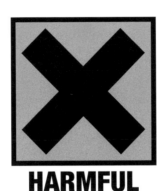
HARMFUL

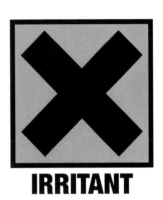
IRRITANT

OXIDISING

HIGHLY FLAMMABLE

TOXIC

Plate: 2.1 Hazard symbols: a collection of some of the common hazard symbols and their meanings often found in biomedical laboratories. This is not an exhaustive list! Hazard symbols reproduced with the kind permission of the Health and Safety Executive Publications Section.

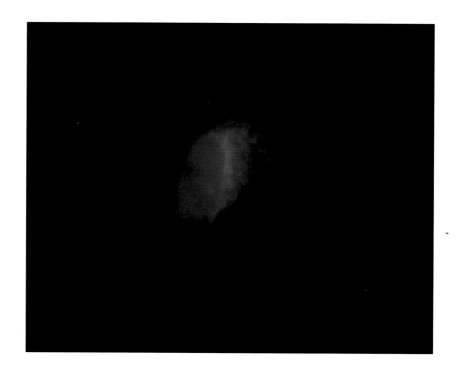

Plate: 8.1 Example of immunofluorescence staining. The image shows immunofluorescence labelling of the microtubules staining in a hTERT-RPE1 cell with
the Alexa 655chromophore. The nucleus is counterstained blue with DAPI
(4',6-diamidino-2-phenylindole). (Image supplied courtesy of Dr Angelo Agathanggelou, Chromatin and Gene Expression Group, Division of Immunology and
Infection, University of Birmingham.)

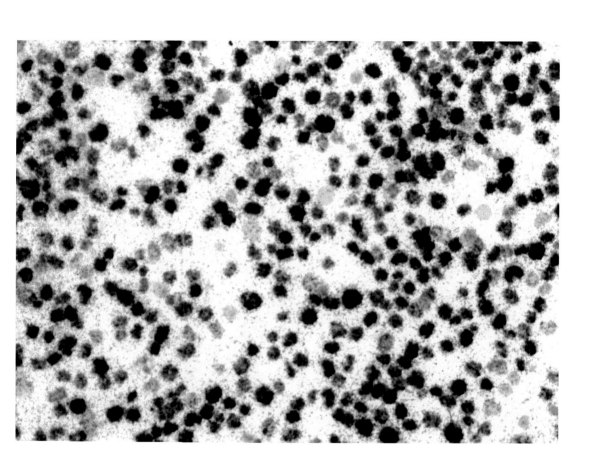

Plate: 8.2 Example of an *in situ* hybridisation using a radiolabelled RNA probe. S^{35}- labelled EBER2 (EBV encoded RNA2) probe was used to show the presence of Epstein-Barr virus (EBV) infection in the lymphoblastoid cell line X50-7. Hybridisation of the radioactive probe is indicated by the deposition of silver grains over the nuclei of the prepared cells, which are counterstained blue with haemotoxylin. (Image supplied courtesy of Dr Angelo Agathanggelou, Chromatin and Gene Expression Group, Division of Immunology and Infection, University of Birmingham.)

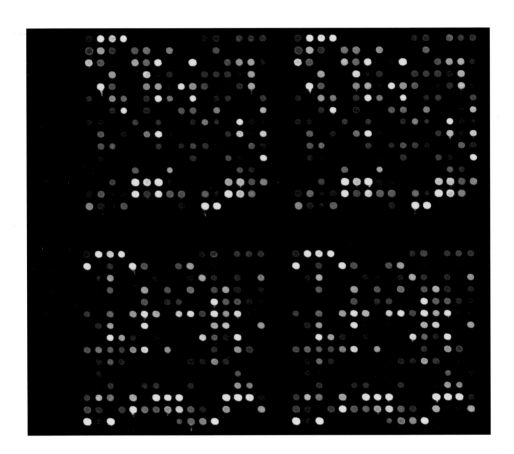

Plate: 10.4 Example of microarray. The image shows a scan of a Leukaemia Research Fund cDNA microarray competitively hybridised with Cy3- (green) and Cy5- (red) labelled cDNAs generated from control and drug-treated HL60 cells. Red and green spots represent genes predominantly expressed in each sample, and yellow spots indicate genes having equal expression levels. (Image supplied courtesy of Mr Vibhor Gupta, Chromatin and Gene Expression Group, Division of Immunology and Infection, University of Birmingham.)

Chapter 6

Scientific writing

What is scientific writing?

Scientific writing is a form of communication that allows the clear and precise dissemination of scientific ideas, empirical data, unique theories and concepts, reviews of previous data and new proofs. This is so that other scientists can judge the soundness of the results presented, and in some cases attempt to validate the findings by reproducing the experimental set-up in other labs. Thus any piece of scientific writing in the biomedical sciences must contain enough practical information for the technique to be copied by an appropriately trained person, and for the robustness and 'believability' of the results to be ascertained.

The style has evolved to contain many 'traditions' or 'correct ways' that are sometimes difficult for the new researcher to emulate. If you are writing your first report, dissertation or thesis, just getting started can be very daunting, especially if you are not sure about the kind of language or approach you need to use.

Generally a piece of scientific writing should be a detailed description of what you have done during your research/project, set in the context of the scientific environment and the current literature on the subject. It should push back the boundaries of understanding even just a little bit further, be it by explaining new discoveries, introducing new techniques or describing refined or improved methodologies. It should always adhere to the style of the publisher you are hoping to use, i.e. if it is to be published by a particular journal, then it should follow the house policy on the number of sections, fonts, referencing system etc. These details vary from journal to journal, but generally the principles are the same.

Most 'papers', as they are often referred to, follow a similar structure. Reading the current literature in your field can help you to familiarise yourself not only with what is happening in your research area, but also the way in which the story is being told. It is easier to start to write your first scientific paper if you have some idea of how others are doing it! To save repetition in this chapter, any kind of scientific writing from a paper for a journal, to a final year dissertation will be referred to as a 'report'.

Basic principles

Most reports are structured to tell the reader the story of what you have done with your research. The detailed breakdown of a report will be considered in a later section, but most styles begin with an introduction to set the scene of the work within the current literature followed by a description of the methods that tell the reader how the experiments were actually done. Next there is a results section describing what was found out as a consequence of those experiments, and a discussion explaining why the results are so important/interesting/worthy of a Nobel prize! This is followed by a conclusion, summing the whole lot up and hinting as to what may come next. This is followed by the possibly dull, but essential references section, and any appendices containing data useful enough to be included, but not interesting enough to put in the other main sections.

As well as deciding what to put into your report, you must also make the important and sometimes difficult decision of what *not* to put in! It should not be a chronological list of all of the experiments that you have performed, even if you have worked in a generally sequential manner. Instead the report should bring together the whole of the story of your discoveries, and this probably means linking together the findings from different experiments from various times in a way that you probably could not have imagined when you set out. Very few 'projects' follow the initial plan exactly – it wouldn't be any fun if they did; and so the job of the report is to bring together all of the fragments of the research jigsaw in such a way as to make the picture complete so that the reader can see what you have achieved, and be inspired by your findings.

Most reports will not contain any information describing mistakes or failures unless they in themselves lead to a new finding or an improvement of a current technique. Certainly experiments that just went wrong because something was spilt or incubated at the wrong temperature should never be included. For a short-term project report, such as that resulting from a final year undergraduate research placement, data can sometimes be scarce, as you may have only spent a few weeks or months in the lab. In these cases some indication of what you actually attempted, even if no solid data were produced, can be very important to show your understanding of the work you undertook, and the amount of effort you have expended! People have received good degrees with very little data, on the back of an excellently written report!

However, for a PhD thesis and for a report which is going to be published in the public domain, the rule holds true: new and robust data leading to new thought-provoking ideas must be present, or there is no point in writing the report.[1]

Planning and more planning

Before you sit yourself down in front of a blank screen, you should spend some time planning what it is you want your report to say. There are various techniques for approaching a 'project' of this kind, but a simple way to start is to ask yourself a basic question – 'what did I do it for?'.

This can then be expanded out into three further questions:

- what was I trying to show?
- what hypothesis was I trying to prove?
- what question(s) was I asking?

The answers to these fundamental queries will help you to formulate your underlying message, and clarify for yourself an overview of what you have done. It is very easy to get bogged down in the details of a scientific report and lose sight of the main message that you want to convey. If that message isn't clear to you from the outset, then you cannot hope to communicate it effectively, and it will certainly not be clear to the reader once the report is finished. These questions should also be reconsidered on completion of the report, to ensure that they have been fully answered!

Once you have made your overarching story clear, then you can move onto more specific questions, such as 'what do I want to say?'. Again this can be expanded into more specific questions:

- what have I found out?
- what new things have I shown?
- what is the bottom line?

The answers to these types of questions will form the basis of your results/ discussion/conclusions sections, as this is where you bring your ideas together into a coherent whole to convince the reader of your discoveries. By now you should have a good idea of what your story is going to be, and have identified some of the key ideas you will need to use to 'tell' that story.

The next step is to consider some of the tools that you may need to make the story detailed enough for scientific readers, while still ensuring that it is fully understandable. To decide what you may need consider 'how can I best explain it?'. This leads you to consider different ways of communicating the data and results:

- what is the best approach to present my data?
- will I need graphs or photographs?
- do I need schemes and diagrams?

The answers to these questions produce a basic list of items that you must produce to incorporate into your report. If you have taken many photographs of microscope slides, or cells in culture, now is the time to decide which are the best ones to include. Choose those that are the clearest and best illustrate the point you are trying to make. With the use of scanners and digital cameras it is much easier (and cheaper) to produce and store many images of this kind over the course of a research project. However you should not try and use them all! Be selective and always have a good reason for including all those you choose to use. Getting multiple images of this kind printed out can sometime be a time-consuming business, so you may want to start the production line early on, so that it can be running alongside your writing and editing, and not come as a big last-minute job as you approach your deadline for completion! In addition if your actual writing hits a brick wall, producing diagrams and photos can be a useful thing to potter on with so that you don't lose momentum, or waste time.

Similarly turning raw numerical data into publication-standard graphs and tables can also take time. You should have been plotting rough working graphs of your data as the research project progressed for inclusion into your lab book, but these will need further work to tidy them up for publication into your report. A quick look at the data at this early stage can help you decide if you are going to use just a few graphs or hundreds, and will help you plan your time accordingly. If you need to produce a complex flow chart or reaction scheme, then you should try to produce some early drafts, which will also help to inform your writing, and give you the chance to think about whether they are the best way to say what you want to say. There is always more than one way to get the message across, so you may consider various approaches before you find the ideal solution.

At this stage you should have lots of ideas about how your project is going to hang together, and a fair idea of what kind of things you need to put into it. You don't want to lose these threads, so a good plan for keeping track of them all is to use a hardbound notebook. This can be a very useful companion to the process of writing a report as it can fulfill many different jobs! Top tips for using the notebook approach are shown in Box 6.1.

Box 6.1   Top tips for using the notebook approach

- Use bound instead of loose-leaf so you don't lose anything, or get them out of order. The chronological order of your entries can be important.
- Jot down ideas for later sections as and when they come to you, so that you don't forget them!
- Use it to keep track of what you have already done and what you need to do next.
- Rewrite your lists as you complete more and more of the sections.
- Don't be afraid to change your plans as you go along; the ideas in the notebook are fluid, not fixed. However you should keep those earlier ideas just in case you want to revert back to a previous version, or re-use them somewhere else.

The notebook can also be used to write your contents planners; start with a basic list of headers you might want to use, as well as those for the graphs, photos and diagrams that you need. As you produce them, cross them off. It can be very encouraging to 'finish' small sections of the report, especially if you feel you aren't making much progress! Another type of 'planner' can be the concept map. Here you expand the basic headers into wider concepts of what you might wish to include. Again these are not fixed in stone; you will certainly want to change them as your writing progresses, but they can be useful to get an idea of the structure of the report and what falls into each part or section. It can also be used to highlight bits of information you will need to know eventually, but do not yet have to hand, such as the name of a supplier for a particular reagent you have used. You don't need to worry about details like that in the early stages, but neither do you want to forget that you need to find out! Figure 6.1 is an example of a diagram like this showing you how it would be used for the general planning of your report, and to keep track of where you are and what you still need to do. The figure shows an example 'concept map' roughing out the basic structure of a scientific report. The main sections are connected 'bubbles', with content suggesting subsections and notes and queries attached. This is a useful way of getting ideas quickly down onto paper without being constrained by formal text.

Starting a report can sometimes be the hardest part (apart from finishing one), but by using the techniques described above; producing concept maps and heading planners, lists of graphs and diagrams, etc, you can clearly define what you are trying to achieve and get a little bit of the

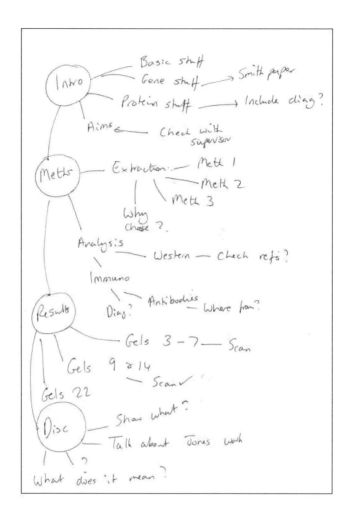

Figure 6.1 Concept map.

'donkey' work out of the way early on. This is a much easier way to make a start and see some progress than by trying to write the first sentence from nothing.

Starting and drafting

Once you do start to write you are into the 'world of drafts'. The first thing you may need to accept is that the first version of anything you write will probably be rubbish! Don't ever expect a section to be perfect (or even just OK) the first time that you write it. What you must keep sight of is that no matter how bad the first draft is, it is much, much nearer to the finished report than a blank page can ever be. It is better to start to get a section written, and to get your ideas down on paper even if they are not fully formulated, or you aren't happy with exactly the turn of phrase you have used. Sometimes you need time for your thoughts to stew in your head for a while, to fully develop and mature into the kind of quality of writing that you need. Getting the early versions recorded can help with that process, and allows you to consider the writing that you have done, in a more objective and critical frame of mind at a later time. Tips for getting on with the first draft are shown in Box 6.2.

Box 6.2   Top tips for getting on with the first draft

- Break it down into small bite-sized chunks that are achievable in a single sitting.
- Work out of sequence if you want to.
- Start with some of the 'easier' sections to make some quick progress and give yourself a boost.
- Leave out tricky sections or minor details to be filled in later – gaps are OK!
- Manage your time carefully – if you are struggling with a section leave it and try another; don't waste all day feeling frustrated and not making progress
- Tick off your list/planner as you complete sections.
- Read your drafts out loud to yourself or to someone else to check the language and the clarity.
- Weaker sections can be revised or amended as you go along.

Once you have written the first draft you can move forward to the second! Remember no matter how bad the first draft may be when you come to read it again, it is always easier to have something to work on and develop, even if none of the actual sentences from the first draft make it into the second! Sometimes reading the first version of what you have written helps you to pick out exactly what it was you wanted to say (and perhaps what it was that you didn't), and enables you to reword the phrase in a much better way. However the second draft probably won't be the last; expect to go through three, four or five drafts – possibly more for difficult sections. Use each iteration to revise, refine and clarify what you are saying – but don't be afraid to throw a section away completely and start from scratch if you feel you have ended up in a dead end, or want to alter the approach. It can be a good idea to save each of these 'versions' separately, both as printed and electronic records of your thought processes. This is very handy if you then decide to go back to a previous way of explaining something! Another good tip is to keep multiple electronic versions in different places, at work and at home, on a disk or data stick. If someone steals your laptop, you don't want to have lost the only version (and I speak from experience!).

Get opinions from your colleagues – after reading a section of your writing can they explain back to you what it said? If they can't, then you need to find out why; which part was difficult to understand or had confusing explanations? Be tough on yourself – does it really say what you want it to say?

Styles and formats

When writing for a scientific journal, there will probably be a house style that you must adhere to. Details of what this consists of can be found in copies of the journal, or via their online 'Instructions to authors'. If you have a particular journal in mind for a paper then it can save you time and effort to begin to write, even from the first draft, in that style. The 'style' of a paper or report is a description of the basic structure, the font used in the printed text, text point size, the type of headings, the page layout and so on. How easily you use these will depend on your level of expertise with word processing packages, but once you decide you will probably find it quicker to work within a 'template', so that every new page or section automatically adheres to that style. Again, further training may save you time.

Choice of fonts

There are many interesting and decorative fonts available even with a standard word processing package, but they are generally not appropriate for use in the scientific report! In the next set of examples, extracts of real and 'doctored' final year reports and papers are used as examples.[2–4]

As you can see from Example 6.1, these types of font do not lend themselves well to scientific clarity; they look wrong and can be quite difficult to read. Generally you are better off sticking to a few standard (if a little boring) 'traditional' fonts such as Times, Palatino or Arial.

Example 6.1[2,3]

AChE Gene and Molecular Forms

The catalytic subunits of AChE appear to arise from a single gene (Taylor & Radic, 1994) mapped to the 7q22 chromosomal position (Ehrlich et al, 1992). Electrophoretic studies of electric organ homogenates revealed the presence of several polymorphic forms of AChE.

Assembly of Molecular Forms
Evidence concerning the assembly of the isoforms is contradictory. Massoulie and Bon (1982) proposed that G forms are degradation products of the more complex A forms. However experiments performed in embryonic rat myotube cultures provided an alternative explanation.

Example 6.2

Palatino

The catalytic subunits of AChE appear to arise from a single gene (Taylor & Radic, 1994) mapped to the 7q22 chromosomal position (Ehrlich *et al*, 1992).

Arial

Electrophoretic studies of electric organ homogenates revealed the presence of several polymorphic forms of AChE. Evidence concerning the assembly of the isoforms is contradictory.

Times New Roman

Massoulie and Bon (1982) proposed that G forms are degradation products of the more complex A forms. However experiments performed in embryonic rat myotube cultures provided an alternative explanation.

Layout

Similarly when considering your layout, you may wish to use left align or perhaps justified paragraphs, with or without initial indents. Watch out if you are using justified, as narrow pages and long words can sometimes lead to an untidy spreading of words over the line, leaving unsightly gaps or 'runs' of white! You may also decide to have your section headings emphasised in some way. Usually this consists of simply making them bold, a slightly larger point size, or using italics. You could of course use all three!

Example 6.3   Align left, header in bold

AChE Gene and Molecular Forms

The catalytic subunits of AChE appear to arise from a single gene (Taylor and Radic, 1994) mapped to the 7q22 chromosomal position (Ehrlich *et al*, 1992). Electrophoretic studies of electric organ homogenates revealed the presence of several polymorphic forms of AChE.

Example 6.4   Justified, header in point 14 and italics

Assembly of Molecular Forms

Evidence concerning the assembly of the isoforms is contradictory. Massoulie and Bon (1982) proposed that G forms are degradation products of the more complex A forms. However experiments performed in embryonic rat myotube cultures provided an alternative explanation.

Another way of structuring your layout is to use a numbering system. This is often used for project reports or PhD theses, and can be very helpful when planning the structure as discussed previously. In this system each major section or 'chapter' is assigned a number, and each subsection is given a number within that number, e.g. 'Chapter 1, Section 5' or '1.5'. This can be invaluable for keeping track of multiple sub, subsections, as theoretically the numbering system will hold forever, potentially giving you section headings such as '1.5.1.1'! Another advantage of this system is that not only will most word processing packages do this automatically (although they can get carried away if you let them) it allows you to easily miss out sections or insert new ones, while not losing sight of where you are. Similarly if you are keeping track of your progress in a notebook, it is easy to monitor your progress by tracking the numbered sections. Thus 'must do 2.4.5 and find graph for 3.3.5' becomes a quick and easy way of maintaining a to-do list, and you always know what part of the report you are referring to.

Example 6.5[4]

1.11 AChE Gene and Molecular Forms

The catalytic subunits of AChE appear to arise from a single gene (Taylor & Radic, 1994) mapped to the 7q22 chromosomal position (Ehrlich *et al*, 1992). Electrophoretic studies of electric organ homogenates revealed the presence of several polymorphic forms of AChE.

1.12 Assembly of Molecular Forms

need to do this section next . . .

1.13 Regulation and Localisation of AChE

After motor nerve section, AChE levels in the muscle decline (Weinberg & Hall, 1979). Proteases released by muscle cells appear to be responsible for the decrease in endplate levels of A forms via proteolysis: Fernadez and Duell (1980) found that administration of protease inhibitors enabled normal levels of enzyme to be maintained after nerve section.

Another advantage of this approach (if you haven't yet been convinced) is the easy way this type of system can be used to make a heading planner and then ultimately your index. It even makes it easy to label figures or graphs! Even if the report you are writing will not ultimately end up being published with the numbers (i.e it's for a journal) it can still be helpful to work like this, and then remove them all at the end once the report is completed.

Example 6.6

Chapter 2 Materials and Methods

2.1	Materials	18
2.11	Buffer solutions	18
2.12	Reagents	
	2.121 Determination of AChE activity	18
	2.122 Determination of β-galactosidase (16S) activity	18
	2.123 Determination of ADH (4.5S) activity	19
2.2	Animals	19
2.21	Treatment	19

Style of writing

Another, perhaps more fundamental consideration of 'style' is not to do with the type of font or paragraph forms. This 'style' is to do with striking the right 'tone' of voice when writing for a scientific audience. Usually this consists of writing in the 'third' person, and the past tense, avoiding any use of the word 'I'. If you have not written in this way before, it can be difficult, and you may find that you slip back to wrong style occasionally. Don't worry; getting the information down onto the paper is much more important at first. You can sort the style and tenses later – that is why you work with multiple drafts!

Consider the next two examples, describing a method. The first is muddled and difficult to follow, and sounds 'amateurish'. The second contains exactly the same information, but is written in a more scientific way, and is much clearer to read and understand, and therefore would be easier to potentially replicate in the lab.

Example 6.7

2.82 Determination of β-galactosidase
To test the enzyme I mixed the buffer, phosphate made up as 0.34 M and pHed to 7.3, with $MgCl_2$ made up at 3 mM and 50 µl of sample and ONPG at 0.28 µM. I had made the sample by layering 100 µl of β-galactosidase made up at 100 units/ml on top of the sucrose gradient as I did before. I took the readings after 5 minutes at 414 nm in the same way. The substrate was added last to begin the reaction.

2.82 Determination of β-galactosidase

A 100 μl sample of β-galactosidase (100 units/ml) was layered on top of a sucrose gradient and centrifuged as described above. The incubation mixture consisted of 0.34 M phosphate buffer (pH 7.3), 3 mM $MgCl_2$, 50 μl of test sample and the substrate, 0.28 μM ONPG. The substrate was added to start the reaction. After 5 minutes the absorbance was read at 414 nm as previously described.

Although past tense is the usual style, present tense is sometimes appropriate, such as in the introduction of your report while describing accepted truths.

Example 6.8

1.1 General Structure and Mechanism of Action

AChE belongs to the family of serine hydrolases. It shows significant sequence homology with other members of the family. The three-dimensional structure of AChE taken from *Torpedo* is shown in Figure 1.1 (Massoulie *et al*, 1993).

When explaining and discussing your findings however, you should generally stick with the past tense, as it is a description of what you *have* done, in the past, over the course of your project.

Example 6.9

3.31 Comparison of Separation Profiles with the Profiles for Marker Enzymes

The activity of β-galactosidase fell between fraction 5 and fraction 10. No peak for A12 activity was observed between these fraction numbers in any of the hearts examined. Figures 3.2 and 3.3 show that the peak for the G4 form of AChE generally fell between fractions 26 and 36, with the optimum slightly to the right of that for alcohol dehydrogenase activity, which separated between fractions 24 and 31.

This also holds for your discussion/conclusions section, although it may be more difficult to do. In some situations such as a review of the current literature an established scientist may use 'I' to express a personal opinion of some data, but this can sound very 'me, me, me' (or I, I, I!) in a report or thesis. Generally staying in the third person here too can help to formalise the arguments and discussions, which will lend weight to your hypothesis.

Example 6.10

First person

I have considered several possible explanations for the relative distribution of AChE in different regions of the heart that I found in this study. Firstly I noticed that although the left atrium does not contain specialised areas, postganglionic innervation may be sufficient for nerve-associated AChE to exceed that of the right atrium.

I also found that the activity of AChE in the left ventricle was higher than that of all other regions including the right ventricle. This means I disagree with the findings of Nyquist-Battie and Trans-Saltzmann (1989).

Third person

There are several possible explanations for the relative distribution of AChE in different regions of the heart found in this study. Firstly although the left atrium does not contain specialised areas, postganglionic innervation may be sufficient for nerve-associated AChE to exceed that of the right atrium.

The activity of AChE in the left ventricle was higher than that of all other regions including the right ventricle. This is in contrast to the findings of Nyquist-Battie and Trans-Saltzmann (1989).

So, general tips for achieving a good scientific style are as shown in Box 6.3.

Box 6.3 Top tips for achieving a good scientific style

- Be clear
- Be concise
- Be consistent
- Choose an appropriate font/layout/style
- Check the grammar, spellings and tenses very carefully
- Don't waffle
- Read it out loud to check for clarity

The structure of scientific papers

Basic structure

Most scientific papers/reports follow a standard structure, which enables the reader to follow a logical progression through the story being told, supplying evidence for all of the statements made and building up to a main point or claim. Individual journals may condense, rearrange or dispense with some of these structures, but most will be used and so it is useful to consider what each section is for. The usual structure is shown in Box 6.4.

Box 6.4   Usual structure for a report

- Abstract or summary
- Introduction
- Methods
- Results
- Discussion
- Conclusion(s)
- References
- Appendices

The abstract or summary

This is a short description of the whole report, briefly describing the aims of the project, the methods used, the main results found and the primary conclusions. It is usually very short, only a page or so of text, and may be regulated down to only 200–250 words in some instances. It should give the reader a good feel for what is in the rest of the report, and hopefully whet their appetite for what is to come! As you know, readers often browse abstracts (sometimes online) and will only bother to read the full paper if the abstract grabs their attention. Writing the abstract is often one of the last sections to tackle, as you cannot realistically describe everything in the report in such a concise way until you have written the rest of the report!

Condensing possibly hundreds of pages down to just one is a challenge, and it certainly tests your ability to be concise! A good approach is to assume that you will write too much initially, and then ferociously prune the text until you get down to your target word count. It you still weren't sure what your report was really saying, then you certainly will be, after you have written the abstract!

The introduction

The introduction is there to give the reader the full scientific background to the project, and should be detailed enough to give a person from outside the field the information that they need to be able to follow and understand the forthcoming data and conclusions. It should include a full review of the pertinent literature, possibly in a chronological manner, but certainly it should build up the reader's understanding of the 'story' right up to the edge of current knowledge – where your findings should take over! This full coverage of the literature must be fully referenced so that the reader can see the source of every statement of fact that you make.

The review must however remain focused; it can be very easy to become sidetracked by interesting papers or ideas, which although they have scientific merit, do not add significantly to your 'story' and may distract or confuse the reader. Every statement that you make should be something that will be useful for the reader to know when reading later parts of the report. You must also remember that you cannot include every single paper on a given topic! Even if your line of research is very unusual or obscure it is still very likely to have thousands of potential papers that you could include. Thus deciding what *not* to include can sometimes be as difficult as deciding what *to* include. Check with your colleagues/supervisor that you have included all of the 'classic' papers in the field, so as not to leave any potentially embarrassing gaping holes, but don't be afraid to include some less well-known papers if they are pertinent to your argument.

The final section of the introduction should be a set of clear aims for your project. These might not end up being the same as those that you started with at the beginning of the project. This is often the case as your developing understanding, greater knowledge of the subject and emerging results inevitably alter your ideas of what you are trying to achieve. Certainly for a final year project or thesis, you must ensure that the aims as described in the introduction are met (more or less) by the following report.

Thus a well-written introduction and aims will enable you to lead the reader by the hand through the literature right up to where it ends, and your research takes over . . .

The methods

The methods chapter may be segregated into separate 'materials' and 'methods' sections, or kept as one 'Methods' chapter; but whichever approach is used it should still contain a concise description of all of the laboratory techniques you have used, and how you have used them. It should not necessarily be in the chronological order in which you learned or utilised the techniques, but should be ordered in a logical fashion, building from the simple preparatory techniques to the more complex multistage methodologies.

It must contain all of the recipes for every reagent used, and the commercial supplier from which they were purchased. It should also contain information describing exactly how that particular reagent or sample was used, for instance what concentration, what temperature, what pH etc. In essence, it should be detailed enough for a competent researcher to be able to pick up and repeat exactly what you have done with no further instruction from you. If you are not sure your written methods are achieving this, then again enlist the help of other colleagues to read the experimental descriptions as though they were going to have a go. If they need to ask you too many questions about how they should proceed, then you need to review what you have written!

Take care when writing text that is full of numerical information, as you can easily lose the odd zero here and there; and make sure that you always include the correct units. If a reagent is particularly complex or has many different components, then describing it in prose may be tedious to read. In this case you could consider moving the details to an adjacent table or materials section at the end of the chapter. As usual check for the regulations on styles for the intended target of your report.

The results

Now we get to the nitty-gritty part of the report! This is the section where you finally get to describe what you have done and what you have found. The results section is a detailed description of the data that you have produced, the slides you have studied and the readings that you took. Here is where you include all of the graphs and tables, photographs, data spreadsheets, statistical analysis and anything else you have used, to produce and illustrate your new findings.

You must take care to organise this plethora of information in a logical manner, so that you build on your story and show how one result leads to the next. However, the results section should have no discussion of what the results might mean; it only includes a description of them. This can be quite difficult, as your mind tends to run on to the implications of a result, as you explain what you have found. If this is the case then you should jot down these ideas as a starter to the first draft of your discussion, if they are helpful. It is often easier to alternate between writing the *results* of an experiment, and writing the *discussion* of what those results may mean while that meaning is still fresh in your head, than to write them completely separately, possibly weeks/months apart! However, whichever way you decide to work, you must have the results of the experiment and associated graphs etc drafted and in front of you before you can seriously address what the implications of those results might be.

The discussion and conclusions

This section is where you describe and explain what your results mean, what they show, and how important they are. They should be set within the context of the current knowledge, so don't be afraid to re-introduce information from the literature that you mentioned in the introduction. Perhaps other papers that you have read, which were not appropriate for the literature review, are now much more useful as they help to shed light on the interpretation of your new findings. Maybe there are some publications that your findings now disagree with!

The discussion section is your chance to show what *you* think is happening, and for you to show that you have added to the sum of knowledge in your field, even if it is only by a little. It should show how you have interpreted the results that you have produced to find a meaning, and it should be full of your new ideas and theories.

The final section of the discussion should be the conclusions. In some journal formats, this is an additional section and not part of the discussion, so again you may need to check the regulations for your report. The conclusion, however it comes, should be the place where you show *your* understanding of what it all means – the bottom-line if you like! It should probably be quite short and punchy and may include a point-by-point listing of how your final suppositions support or challenge your initial hypothesis. You may then want to mention a few ideas expounding on what should be done next; a little taster, maybe, of how the research you have done may be developed further.

The references and appendices

If you are to properly refer to every source of information that you used in order to write your report (and this is not optional, you *must* do this), then you should try to do two things from the very start of the writing process. The first is to keep a very close track of all of those sources as and when you use them; and the second is to make sure that every time you use them to make a point or back up an argument, they are properly cited. There are two standard systems used by most scientific reports (*see* later) and different journals may favour one over the other. The key point that you must remember is that a reader must be able to use the system to find the details of that paper in the list of references, and then be able to find the full paper themselves, if they so wish. Further information on referencing systems is given in the next section. Failure to cite correctly can be considered to be plagiarism, as it implies that you are not crediting the original author for their work, and it may be inferred that you are claiming it as an idea of your own. This is a serious consideration for final year projects and PhD theses, as well as papers being submitted for publication in peer-reviewed journals.

The final section in a report may be the appendices. These are not always needed but can be used to house quantities of data, additional graphs, multiple photographs etc which, while important to the project as a whole, are not pertinent enough to the story to be used in the main text. It may be that a summary table is used in the results section, but that it is useful to provide access to the contributing data to that table for those who may be interested, or who want to be sure you are not making too many inferences from your data!

Referencing systems

The first system commonly in use is the 'Vancouver', which uses a numerical approach to track citations. With this system, every time a statement is made which uses a particular text as a source, a small superscripted number is placed at the end of the sentence. The list of references is then built up by listing these texts against their descriptive number. If a text or paper is referred to again later on, it still retains the first number that it was given. The numerical listing starts with the first reference and goes on up. This can create difficulties if, at a later time or in a subsequent draft, an additional reference is included, as all those that come later will consequently need to change their number by one! An example of the Vancouver system is shown in Box 6.5.

Box 6.5   The Vancouver system

Text

Although early studies in the rat showed that the cholinergic innervation on the ventricle is sparse,[21] electron microscopy of the ventricular muscle of the dog has revealed the prescence of cholinergic nerve endings.[22] Furthermore, radioligand binding studies[23] have revealed . . .

References

21 Levy MN. Parasympathetic control of the heart. In: WC Randall (ed.) *Neural Regulation of the Heart*. New York: Oxford University Press; 1975, pp. 95–129.

22 Yamauchi A. Ultrastructure of the innervation of the mammalian heart. In: CE Challice and Viragh S (eds) *Ultrastructure of the Mammalian Heart*. New York: Academic Press; 1973.

23 Yang CM, Yeh HM, Sung TC, Chen FF and Wang YY. Characterisation of muscarinic receptor subtypes in canine left ventricular membranes. *Journal of Receptor Research* 1992; 12: 427–49.

The other commonly used system is the Harvard. This uses the actual names of authors and dates of publication in the text, either contained in parentheses or as part of the prose. The list of references is then built up in alphabetical order of lead author. This system can be easier to use when first writing, as having the names of the authors present in the text may help to remind you of the details of the paper you have sourced. It is also easier to add extra citations as this only requires an insertion at the correct point of the list. An example of the Harvard system is shown in Box 6.6.

Box 6.6   The Harvard system

Text

. . . as shown by other workers (Ghosh *et al.*,1991; Goodwin and Sizer, 1965), or via increased expression of POMC-derived neurotropic peptides or other peptides which have been shown to regulate ACHE levels (Amos and Smith, 1998) . . .

References

Amos ML and Smith ME. The effect of pyridostigmine administration on the expression of POMC-derived peptides in motoneurons. *Neurotoxicology* 1998; 19: 799–808.

Ghosh P, Bhattacharya S and Bhattacharya S. Does acetylcholine induce the synthesis of inhibited ACHE in fish brain? In: J Massoulie, E Barnard, A Chatonnet *et al.* (eds) *Cholinesterases*. Washington DC: American Chemical Society; 1991, p. 270.

Goodwin BC and Sizer IW. Effects of spinal cord substrate on acetylcholinesterase in chick embryonic skeletal muscle. *Developmental Biology* 1965; 11: 136–53.

Keeping track of references and typing them into a report in the correct format can be tedious, so try to build your reference list as you go along, again to prevent it becoming a huge job at the end. Make use of an automated system if you can as these can save a lot of time and effort. Examples of these are 'Reference manager' or 'Endnote', and often references downloaded from the web or e-journals can be automatically inserted into these dedicated databases. This avoids problems with mis-spelling unfamiliar names, or errors transcribing the journal volume or page number – all mistakes which are easily made, but which must not happen!

Finishing the report

Next to beginning, finishing the report can sometimes be the hardest part! As each of your sections or chapters progress through their various drafting stages, the whole report slowly begins to come together, and the end is in sight. At this point you may find you have lots of bits and pieces left to do; the odd graph here, or a paragraph you are still not entirely happy with, that diagram that always prints badly. It is easy to falter at this stage as the repeated revisions or minor changes can become a muddled mess, and you can easily get lost in different versions of sections. As you reach this stage you must build in time to *stop*, review the work, and decide where you are and what is still left to be finished. Colleagues may be involved in producing some of the items that you need for the report, such as photos, and so you may be left waiting for them, and unable to sign off sections because of their delays. If you are using a notebook to track your work, then this is when it becomes even more useful as you can identify and record the missing parts and not forget them! You should also try to read larger sections such as a whole chapter in one go, to check that the tone or style is consistent across the whole report, and check that you haven't repeated yourself.

When you write different sections separately, possibly months apart, you can sometimes lose track of what it was you were trying to say. Some sections may work when looked at on their own but need to be rethought when looked at closely within the context of the rest of the report. As well as checking the consistency of the content, you may need to take another look at the layout, and the style of the report. Now that you know what it is that you want to say for a particular part, you may decide that it would be better placed before or after another section.

Once all these final revisions have been completed and all of the graphs/table/photos etc have been produced and collated, it is time to start printing! Publishers for journals sometimes expect to receive hard copies of proposed papers, but much more prevalent now is the online submission route. This will save you time (and trees – some journals used to ask for 10 or more copies of the submission!) but always make sure you have a hard copy for yourself, for quick reference, and in case there is ever a problem with your multiple-copied (backed up everywhere and kept in different buildings in case of theft or fire) electronic version.

If the report is a PhD thesis or final year dissertation, then you will most likely be expected to sort out the printing of this yourself. Do not under-estimate the time that this may take! Printers, as we all know, are temperamental at the best of times, so always have a back up plan if your first choice, either at home or in your institution, decides to have a bad day! Lots of extra ink cartridges are also a very good idea. Even if you have no major mishaps, it may take more than a couple of days to print out successfully multiple copies of a possible 200+ pages of text with colour figures or photos, and then get the report bound in some way. If you are working to a deadline make sure you cost this time in, and don't assume it's a five-minute job!

It can be very hard sometimes to let go of a report that may have been a major undertaking. A PhD thesis may very well have been your *complete life* for 3 or 4 years! This means that you can easily get into the frame of mind where you keep on correcting and redrafting over and over, possibly making very little actual progress or any significant changes. Never being entirely happy with a section can lead you to a position where you will never finish. Some excellent research never sees the light of day, not because it wasn't good enough, but because the author couldn't let it go!

If you have a to work to a deadline, either to hand in the dissertation or thesis, or to meet the publisher's time frame, then you have to be strict with yourself. It may be that the section will never be perfect – but what is? For assessed work you must not allow yourself to lose marks by submitting the work late, just because you are still making minute tweaks and alterations. Remember that being penalised in this way will have a much greater impact on your overall mark than a couple of awkward sentences could ever have!

When submitting new research to be published in journals, there may be an even more pressing time element – competition from other labs! Although we like to think of the scientific community working together to push back the boundaries of understanding, you wouldn't want delays in sending results to the journal to end in your lab being scooped on a new discovery. You may have done it first, but until it's published and out there, no-one will know that you have done it. Obviously you shouldn't rush out your draft papers without proper checks on the quality of the results and the writing. The reviewers will reject good data that is badly written just as easily as bad data. But just be aware that you may need to reach a point where you 'let go' of the writing and allow it to be judged by others. You may need to set a time deadline for changes, or a limit on the number of iterations, but whichever way you do it, make sure that you are still in control and are deciding that it is completed rather than having that decision forced on you by the looming submission date.

References

1   Mathews JR, Bowdem JM and Mathews RW. *Successful Scientific Writing* (2e). Cambridge: Cambridge University Press; 2000.
2   Gill DS, Lintern MC, Wetherell J *et al.* Guinea-pig heart acetylcholinesterase after continuous physostigmine administration. *Human and Experimental Toxicology* 2003; 22: 373–81.
3   Gill DS. Acetylcholinesterase levels in the heart. Submitted as Final Year Research Project, University of Birmingham; 2000.
4   Lintern MC, Wetherell J, Taylor C *et al.* The effect of continuous pyridostigmine administration on functional (A12) acetylcholinesterase activity in guinea-pig muscles. *Neurotoxicology* 2001; 22: 787–93.

Section 2

Biomedical techniques

Chapter 7

Protein techniques

Background on proteins

Proteins are one of, if not the most important group of biological molecules. From different combinations of a set of only 20 amino acids, proteins come in all shapes and sizes and perform many essential jobs such as acting as enzymes to biological reactions, providing mechanical support for cells, participating in the communications between nerve cells or producing motion as seen in muscle cells. Altering the sequence in which these 20 amino acid building blocks are linked provides this enormous diversity of function. This sequence is of course itself dictated by the sequence of the cells' DNA; in other words, the genes. Thus the information contained in every gene is a 'blue print' for a protein and only becomes useful once it is expressed and results in the production of that functioning protein.

The sequence (or *primary* structure) of the amino acids dictates the structure of the chain itself; physical properties such as the size of the side chain or the angle of rotation around the bonds between the amino acids results in folding into regular structures such as the rod-like α-helix or the flat β-pleated sheet. Combinations of these secondary structural formations, along with turns and folds, results in a tertiary structure where individual amino acids distant from each other along the linear sequence may be situated very close to one another, and be able to interact with each other via disulphide links between two cysteine residues. Some proteins consist of more than one polypeptide chain of this sort, and the interactions and spatial arrangement of these multiple chains results in quaternary structures. The interaction between the amino acids in the three-dimensional structure confers biological functionality to the protein, and is referred to as the conformation. Changes to the conformation of a protein can change its functionality, allowing it to begin work as an enzyme, to function as a molecular switch such as a cell membrane receptor, or even to initiate a power stroke as in the contraction of muscle fibres.

This basic understanding of the nature of proteins is very important when you begin to handle them in a laboratory situation. Environments that affect the tertiary or quaternary structures may disable the functionality of the protein; treatments that you use may destroy the secondary or even primary structures. For some investigative techniques this may be exactly what you need to do to study the protein, but you should always understand what the consequences of your actions might be. Many proteins are very heat sensitive and begin to denature or lose this complex structure if left lying about on the lab bench at room temperature for any length of time. As previously explained, all functionality depends on the three-dimensional structure being maintained, and even small alterations in structure may affect an area of significance such as the active site of an enzyme, rendering it incapacitated. Thus any preparatory bench work using proteins, be they enzymes or tissues extracts, should usually be conducted on ice until you are actually ready to study the functionality. It can therefore be very useful to determine how heat labile your protein of interest is, and this information can then be used to decide how carefully you need to treat it!

Another 'property' of any protein is its inherent charge, a factor again dictated by the primary sequence. The individual charges arising from the amino acids culminate in a net charge across the whole protein. This is a property that can be used to help investigate the nature of the protein more fully, and is exploited using techniques like electrophoresis. Once again, however, it results in a range of sensitivities to the pH of the environment, which you may have to consider. This is discussed in more detail when considering enzymes in the next section.[1]

Enzymes

An enzyme is a specialised protein that can perform a biological 'job' such as sticking two molecular elements together or breaking them apart. The presence of an enzyme catalyses the reaction and thus greatly increases the speed that this reaction will occur at, sometimes from effectively zero (i.e. never!) to many thousands of reactions per second. An example of a standard enzyme reaction is shown in Box 7.1.

Box 7.1 Example of a standard enzyme reaction

enzyme

Substrate A + Substrate B ⇔ Product C + Product D

One of the fastest enzymes known is acetylcholinesterase, which degrades the neurotransmitter acetylcholine at neuromuscular junctions, and cholinergic brain synapses. This enzyme must very quickly clear the transmitter from the cleft between the cells after the signal has been carried, so that another signal may be sent in very quick succession.

An enzyme has a complex three-dimensional shape, which is dictated by the primary sequence and the secondary structures such as α-sheets and β-pleats as previously described. These shapes fit together to form a molecule with distinct areas that function as binding sites, active sites and peripheral sites. This functionality is therefore solely an operation of the structure, and the complex as a whole confers the activity of the enzyme.

Many biomedical experiments require a basic understanding of the practical use of enzymes, even if they are being used as tools rather than as the subject of the investigation. For example restriction enzymes that are used to cleave specific DNA sequences are absolutely essential for any kind of research using molecular biology techniques. Enzymes can be fussy, and for them to work efficiently in the way that you want, you need to treat them properly and give them what they want! This means that you need to manipulate the conditions that they are working in to make them as 'happy' as you can. The 'speed' at which an enzyme does its job is usually referred to as the *rate*, and many things can affect this. Enzyme kinetics is a complex subject beyond the remit of this text, but we can consider some of the basic ideas that will act as a starting point to help your experimental design when it comes to considering and using enzymes.[1]

Conditions that enzymes are sensitive to do vary for individual enzymes but for most there is a general set you should consider.

Temperature

Most enzymes work most efficiently at the temperature they were found at 'in the wild'. Thus many run best at 37°C, body temperature for most animals. Generally the warmer an enzyme is, the faster it will work, up to its maximum. You must remember that an enzyme is still a protein, and so if the temperature gets too high then the protein structure will begin to denature, the activity will be lost and your enzyme will be cooked! Some enzymes are sourced from exotic bacteria living around thermal vents; these are used in PCR, making copies of DNA sequences and work most efficiently at 70°C+! For most enzymes the relationship between the rate at which the reaction proceeds and the temperature can be approximated to a linear relationship; in other words if you know the rate for two temperatures, you can construct an equation and predict what the rate will be at other temperatures. Many other factors do have an influence, such as energy states or collision rates, but a general tip is, once you have your enzyme working well at a particular temperature you should probably keep it the same.

pH

Most enzymes will have a range of [H^+] that they are happy to work in; for some this will be very narrow, others are less fussy. However some types of reactions are particularly sensitive to change in pH and will only function close to their optimum pH. If H^+ is a substrate or product of the reaction, then the pH of the environment will alter as the reaction proceeds, which may then affect the rate. Depending on the equilibrium of the reaction this may mean that the reaction proceeds faster and faster, or that it grinds to a halt completely. If you are studying the reaction in a whole cell, the situation is complicated further by the possible buffering of any H^+ present or the subsequent use of the products for reactions further along a biological pathway. Thus you must consider if/how the pH is going to change over the course of the reaction proceeding, and buffer the system appropriately to ensure that it continues in the way that you want.

Substrate availability

If an enzyme uses substrate A and B to make product C, and it then runs out of A, it cannot make any more C! In fact the rate (v) of the reaction (if all other conditions remain the same) varies with the concentration of the substrate. If this is measured experimentally we find that at low concentrations of substrate the relationship is proportional (i.e. linear), and at high concentrations of substrate the rate reaches its maximum and then becomes 'independent' of the concentration of substrate, as long as this remains at this excess or 'saturated' level. This gives us the classic rectangular hyperbola plot of rate reaction against substrate concentration (*see* Figure 7.1). Thus if you want a reaction to proceed at its maximum rate (V_{max}) then you must provide an excess of the substrate(s) for this to occur. If the concentration of the substrate starts to fall below this saturation point, then the rate will fall also. For situations where you are interested in measuring the amount of an active enzyme that is present in the system, it is imperative to maintain an excess of substrate so that the reaction proceeds at its maximum throughout the measurement period. In this way you can measure the amount of substrate that is used up, or more usually the amount of product that is produced, and use this information to calculate the amount or 'units' of enzyme present and

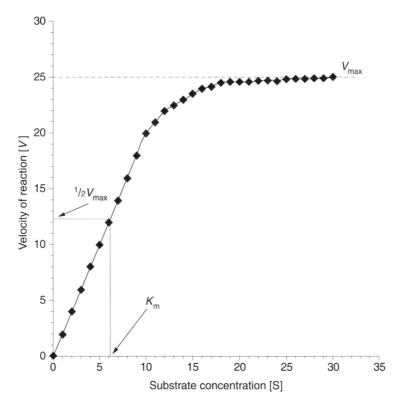

Figure 7.1 Enzyme reaction velocity versus substrate concentration. Plot of the rate of an enzyme reaction v against the concentration of substrate available, showing the classic rectangular hyperbola. V_{max} is the fastest the reaction can proceed at, even with an excess of substrate, but it can be difficult to estimate accurately. K_m is the concentration of substrate at which the reaction proceeds at half its maximum, $\frac{1}{2}V_{max}$. This is the basis of the Michaelis–Menten equation, which is used for studying the kinetics of enzyme catalysed reactions.

working. If there isn't enough substrate for the enzyme to work on, the situation is often referred to as 'substrate limiting'.[2]

In many systems it is very difficult to measure the rate of activity of an enzyme because the amount of product present is hard to measure. Often a 'coupling' reaction is used which enters the product of the first reaction as the substrate of a second reaction. This second reaction results in a product that *can* be easily assessed, for instance one that is strongly coloured. My favourite reaction of this kind, which I have used a lot, is the classic 'Ellman reaction',[3] used for measuring acetylcholinesterase activity, as shown in Box 7.2. The rate of production of the yellow colour can be followed using a spectrophotometer giving an indication of the amount of acetylcholinesterase present.

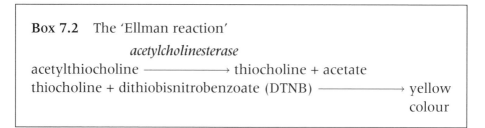

Box 7.2   The 'Ellman reaction'

$$\text{acetylthiocholine} \xrightarrow{\text{acetylcholinesterase}} \text{thiocholine} + \text{acetate}$$

$$\text{thiocholine} + \text{dithiobisnitrobenzoate (DTNB)} \longrightarrow \text{yellow colour}$$

Western blotting

Immuno-blotting or *western* blotting as it is colloquially known (an extension of the *Southern* blotting concept – *see* Chapter 10) is a technique that allows a specific protein of interest to be identified from a mix of other proteins. It relies on the ability of antibodies (proteins themselves, of course) to have a specific affinity for a particular entity, or *antigen*. Thus if protein X is introduced to an animal, the animal recognises it as a foreign body and raises an antibody specific to that protein. If the antibody is then collected from the serum it can be used to pick out protein X from among many other proteins. Antibodies can be so specific that proteins that differ by just a few residues may be differentiated, allowing whole families of very similar proteins to be categorised and their functions studied. For any western blotting technique to yield viable results there are many parameters that must be optimised from a range of possible conditions. Thus no two protocols are ever exactly alike, as they must take into account the affinities of the primary antibody, and the level of target antigen in the sample used, as well as other factors such as the secondary antibody and the detection system used. Thus you may start from a standard lab method but you will always need to vary the conditions to get the best possible (or any) result for your particular antibody on your particular sample. The basic protocol is illustrated in Figure 7.2.

In western blotting, the samples to be analysed are separated on a vertical polyacrylamide gel placed within an electrical field. This is usually abbreviated to PAGE – polyacrylamide gel electrophoresis. Samples of blood, urine, or cellular extracts are prepared in such a way as to denature the protein by boiling in the presence of an ionic detergent such as sodium dodecyl sulphate (SDS) to disrupt the non-covalent interactions. SDS is sometimes called sodium lauryl sulphate; something to remember when hunting for the stock tub on the lab store shelves! The disulphide bonds between the cysteine residues are reduced by β-mercaptoethanol, allowing the protein to unfold. The denatured sample is then usually mixed

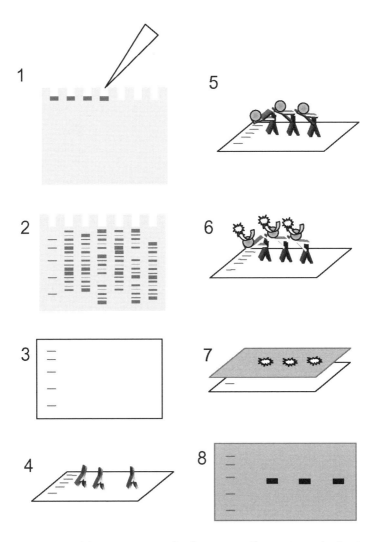

Figure 7.2 Western blotting protocol schematic. Illustration of a basic western blotting protocol showing (1) loading of the prepared protein sample into the wells; (2) separation of the different-sized proteins after electrophoresis. Bands are illustrative only – you would only see the dye front; (3) separated proteins are transferred onto a nylon membrane. If coloured markers are used these can be used to check that the transfer has been successful; (4) the primary antibody binds to the target protein wherever it occurs on the membrane; (5) the secondary antibody binds to the primary antibody. The secondary has a 'marker' molecule such as an enzyme conjugated to it; (6) the enzyme con- jugated onto the secondary antibody reacts with its substrate and produces a light product; (7) the membrane is exposed to hyperfilm, which reacts to the light produced; (8) once developed, the hyperfilm shows a dark band wherever the target protein occurred. The markers help to calibrate the gel and confirm the mass of the target protein.

with a dye such as bromophenol blue so that the progress of the samples can be monitored during the migration.

The large negative charge from the bound SDS makes the charge of the target protein irrelevant, and thus the separation is achieved solely on the basis of the mass of the protein. In essence, the smaller the protein, the further through the gel it will run. Separation is usually performed alongside a 'marker'; a protein or set of proteins of known mass which can be used to calibrate the gel and thus identify the size of the target protein. Markers may be produced in-house, or purchased ready to use from biochemical suppliers. Some even come in a range of colours for easy identification. Depending on the size of the target protein, the size of the cross-links of the gel may be altered. This is easily achieved by changing the percentage of acrylamide in the gel mix. Thus a '15%' gel would have more acrylamide and thus a smaller pore size than a '7%' gel, and would be used for resolving smaller proteins. The resolution or how clearly you can separate and identify similar-sized proteins can also be altered in this way to suit what you want to do. It is therefore helpful when designing and optimising a western blotting system that you have a vague idea how big the protein you want to study is. If your protein is something really new, you might not have any idea at all of the possible size. In this situation the best approach would be to start with a middle-sized gel (maybe 10%) and see where your protein resolves to, which will give a rough idea of its size. You can then alter the gel makeup to improve the resolution.

Once separated through the gel, the proteins are transferred onto a solid support structure so that they can be probed by the antibody. The most common support used is a nylon membrane; this is tough enough to put up with various probing and washing regimes without falling apart, while maintaining the integrity of the transferred proteins. The transfer of proteins from the gel to the membrane constitutes the 'blotting' part of the process, and is usually performed wet with the gel mounted next the membrane and with a current passing through from the gel to the membrane. The positive charge of the membrane prevents any proteins from passing straight through, and so they remain bound to the membrane ready for the probing stage.

At this point many protocols use a blocking step. A wash in a mix of non-fat milk proteins 'blocks' many of the non-specific binding sites similar enough to the target antigen for the primary antibody to stick to them. This improves the level of specific binding. Again it is part of the process of optimisation that will dictate the level, if any, of blocking that you need to use for your antibody with a particular set of target proteins.

The primary antibody, which has a high affinity for your target protein, is now used to probe the membrane. It will bind to wherever it encounters the antigen it recognises – or something similar to it if the affinity is not high enough! This stage may be performed in an incubator at 37°C or room temperature, or overnight at 4°C. Once bound, any non-bound excess primary antibody is removed by washing stages. Primary antibodies can be used at a range of concentrations from 1/50 or 1/100 at the most concentrated end of the scale, to 1/20 000–1/50 000 for those with a very high affinity. Generally you should be aiming to use as low a concentration as possible, but one that still gives you good results. This makes financial sense, but also reduces the levels of 'background' resulting from inappropriate binding to non-specific sites.

The next step is the identification of the primary antibody by a conjugated secondary. The secondary antibody has been raised to recognise any antibody from the animal the primary was raised in. In other words, if your primary was produced in a mouse antibody, then you would need an anti-mouse secondary to recognise and bind to that primary. Attached or conjugated to the secondary is a molecular 'tag' that labels that secondary, and allows its position on the membrane to be identified. This may be a radioactive tag, but more often it will be an enzyme such as hydrogen peroxidase, and again washing the membrane removes any non-specific binding of the secondary to the membrane or the bound proteins. Secondary antibodies are usually much cheaper than primary antibodies, and by choosing a panel of primaries originating from the same host animal, you may be able to use the same secondary for more than one western protocol.

When the enzyme conjugated onto the secondary antibody is provided with its substrates, it mediates a reaction which produces a coloured precipitate or a flash of light. In the latter case the chemiluminescent reaction produces a light that is very faint, and so it is detected by exposing the membrane to a very sensitive film (hyperfilm). What you end up with is a dark band on the hyperfilm identifying your target protein from all the rest of the proteins in the sample, telling you how big it is and in some cases giving an idea of how much is there.

The power of the western blot is the sensitivity of the technique to pick out very low levels of the target protein from a homogeneous mix of many others. This can be used for isolation and further purification of that protein, or simply to decide if it is present or not. When combined with molecular biology techniques, such a when a gene has been introduced to a cell, a western blot will identify the cells that can/are able to express the gene and produce the complete protein.

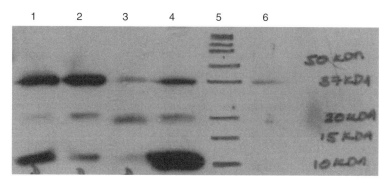

Figure 7.3 Example of a western blot hyperfilm. This example of a western blot hyperfilm shows the marker bands, which have been drawn on in lane 5 and different tissue samples in lanes 1, 2, 3, 4 and 6. The size of the proteins can be calculated from the marker, as these are of known sizes. The relative size and intensity of the band gives a semi-quantitative indication of the amount of the target protein present, assuming the same quantity of total protein was loaded into each lane. Lane 1 shows a strong positive for the 37 kDa and 10 kDa proteins, but not the 20 kDa protein. Lanes 2, 3 and 4 however do show a small amount of the 20 kDa protein. The sample in lane 6 only shows a faint band at 37 kDa. In this way a profile of which proteins (targeted by the primary used in this western blot) are present in each different tissue sample can be built up. (Western blot image reproduced by kind permission of Dr Anna Rowe, Department of Physiology, University of Birmingham.)

Western blotting is common procedure routinely used in many labs. It can be somewhat tedious to work up from scratch with a new set of antibodies for a new target, as every stage can be performed under a range of conditions. Thus, optimising the procedure can be time consuming and requires a systematic approach. However once you have the protocol cracked, it is a very reliable and reproducible system for investigating proteins extracted from cells or tissues. Figure 7.3 is an example of a western blotting hyperfilm.

Proteins can also be separated via electrophoresis on the basis of their charge, which is a result of their acid and basic residues. Using both size separation and isoelectric focusing, a mix of proteins can be separated in two dimensions, and then further investigated. Thus western blotting is only one of many techniques exploiting the chemical properties of proteins in order for us to further investigate their roles in biological systems.

ELISA

The ELISA or 'enzyme-linked immunosorbent assay' technique is very similar to western blotting in so much as it also uses the specificity of

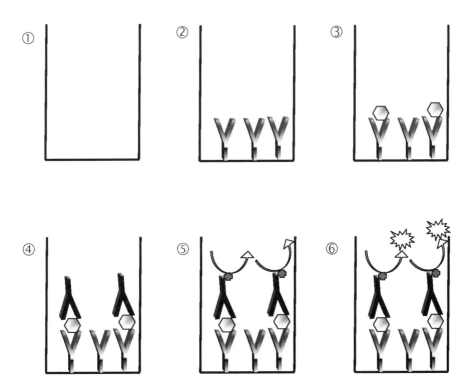

Figure 7.4 ELISA protocol schematic. (1) A 96-well plate is taken and (2) treated with the primary antibody which sticks to the bottom of the plate. The sample to be studied is added to the well, and any target antigen it contains binds to the antibody (3) and other molecules are washed away. A secondary antibody (4) which recognises a different antigenic site is added to the well and binds to the target molecule. This antibody is conjugated to (usually) an enzyme which catalyses a reaction (5). The reaction produces either a coloured product or a flash of light (6) which can be measured. The amount of product gives a quantitative measurement of the amount of target molecule present in the sample in the well. Comparisons can therefore be easily made between many samples in a standard and easily automated procedure.

antibodies to recognise the antigenic site on the target protein. In this system the mix of proteins is not separated by electrophoresis; therefore an ELISA can tell you nothing about the size of your protein, but it can give a semi-quantitative idea of how much is there.

The primary antibody is fixed to a solid support, usually the base of a microtitre plate, and then the mix of proteins is added to the well. Subsequent washes remove all of the proteins, *except* those presenting the antigen recognised by the primary antibody. A secondary antibody, which has been raised against a different antigenic site on the target protein, is then added. This binds to the target protein, which is immobilised by its attachment to the primary antibody. Often multiple secondary antibodies bind to the target, amplifying the signal. The secondary antibody, as in the western system, has a conjugated enzyme that produces a coloured or a highly fluorescent product, which can then be easily detected. Once standardised, ELISA systems are very robust and the solid phase system of microtitre plates allows for a large automated throughput, and makes them ideal for medical diagnostic use. A basic ELISA technique is illustrated in Figure 7.4.

ELISA tests are generally considered to be reliable and accurate and can be made robust enough for use by non-trained persons. An example of this are the over-the-counter pregnancy tests which measure the levels of human chorionic gonadotrophin hormone (HCG) which is produced by the mother very early in the pregnancy and which is excreted in urine. It is measured in these tests using a type of ELISA set up on a simple dipstick.

An alternative use for the ELISA is to measure the presence and levels of a particular antibody of interest, by coating the base of the plate with the antigen. This approach is used to check for HIV antibodies in human serum.

References

1   Stryer L. *Biochemistry* (3e). New York: Freeman and Co; 1989.
2   Morris JG. *A Biologist's Physical Chemistry* (2e). London: Edward Arnold; 1974.
3   Ellman GL, Courtney KD, Andres V Jr and Featherstone RM. A new and rapid colorimetric determination of acetylcholinesterase activity. *Biochemical Pharmacology* 1961; 7: 88–90.

Histological approaches

Co-written with Dr Angelo Agathanggelou.

What is histology?

Techniques such as Southern, western and northern blotting as well as the PCR-based methods can be applied to whole tissue extracts. However, unlike cultured cells, tissue samples are often a heterogeneous mix of cell types. Hence, a possible drawback of using these methodologies is the inability to discriminate between the cell types being analysed. This is the major strength of histological techniques such as immunostaining and *in situ* hybridisation, which can be used to demonstrate the expression of antigens and nucleic acids, respectively, at the cellular level, and their associations with particular cells.

Preparing samples from cell lines

Cells grown in culture need to be put onto glass slides in order for them to be processed for exploratory techniques such as *in situ* hybridisation or immunostaining. The method used depends on whether the cells are adherent (e.g. epithelial cells which like to grow attached to the dish or flask) or in suspension (e.g. lymphoid cells which grow floating around in the media). Cells grown in suspension can be applied to glass slides either by simply dropping small volumes of the suspension onto the slide and hoping they stick, or by using a 'cytospin' centrifuge which places the cell sample more precisely onto the slide, using centripetal force. The same methods can also be used for adherent cells; however these can also be grown directly onto the histological slides. This has the advantage of preserving the cell morphology, which may be of interest to your study. Once cells are on the glass slide, they can be fixed in a manner appropriate to the technique to be used.

Preparing samples from tissues

Tissue samples are normally available in two forms: fixed paraffin embedded and freshly (snap) frozen. Essentially the method for preparation of both types of histological slides is the same, in so much as the original chunks of tissue (e.g. muscle biopsy or brain slice) need be cut into very, very thin sections. Paraffin sections are cut using a microtome, a piece of equipment that uses a very sharp blade (sometimes a type of 'razor blade') to shave very thin slices off the tissue block. These slices or sections, as they are usually referred to, are then floated onto the surface of warm water using a small water bath. The warmth helps to soften the wax slightly, and unwrinkles and unrolls the sections ready for them to be picked up onto a glass slide.

Frozen sections are cut on a 'cryostat' which is essentially the same as a microtome, except that it is enclosed within a freezer unit, which maintains the temperature of the tissue block and the cutting blade at sub-zero temperatures, usually below $-20°C$. The sections are then lifted on to the glass slide, where they thaw and stick. The slides are then usually dried, by exposure to the air or sometimes in an oven. Depending on how they are then going to be used, the process of fixing will vary.

Fixing fresh sections

What does 'fixing' mean? A simple definition of fixing is the process of putting the cryosections or cytological preparations through a treatment regime, which preserves morphological and molecular integrity. The type of fixation used depends again on the technique to be applied, and how roughly you may need to treat the slides! For example, fixation with formaldehyde is required for *in situ* hybridisation-based techniques, because this preserves not only the morphology, but also the nucleic acids. For immunohistology, fixation with solvents such as ethanol, acetone or combinations such as acetone/methanol are favoured. Formaldehyde fixation can also be appropriate, but sometimes the cross-linking is too severe and may mask or denature the antigenic sites. Thus the fixation technique chosen must be considered within the context of the final use of the slides, and the protocol optimised accordingly.

Immunostaining

Once you have your sections cut and fixed, it's time to stain them! There are a number of strategies, which can be largely categorised into two basic methods: immunohistochemistry and immunofluorescence. The general principles for both methods are the same. Step 1 is to expose the prepared section to the primary antibody for the required target antigen. Step 2 uses a conjugated secondary antibody that binds to the primary antibody. The conjugate on the secondary antibody can be either an enzyme (immu-nohistochemistry) or a fluorescent marker (immunofluorescence).

Immunohistochemistry localises an enzyme (e.g. horseradish perox-idase (HRP) or alkaline phosphatase (AP)) to the target antigenic site of interest. The section is then incubated in a substrate solution specific for the enzyme used, and a coloured precipitate is produced where the antibody is bound, indicating the presence of the target molecule. An ordinary light microscope can be used to look at the results of the stained sections. Immunohistochemistry can be used to distinguish nuclear, cytoplasmic and membrane (plasma and nuclear) antigens.

Immunofluorescence differs from immunohistochemistry in that the conjugated label is visualised directly using a UV microscope. A wide range of different labels are commercially available, giving you myriad of colours to choose from! Examples include FITC (fluorescein isothiocya-nate), which fluoresces green, and Texas Red, which is, unsurprisingly, red. The advantage of using the fluorescent system is that a higher level of resolution is achievable. Immunofluorescence allows for the detection of individual organelles such as mitochondria, nucleoli, Golgi bodies, cen-trioles, cytoskeletal elements (actin fibres, microtubules) and even chro-mosomes . . . . Another advantage is that it allows for the simultaneous detection of more than one antigen within the same cell. For this to work the primary antibodies used should either be raised in different animals (e.g. rabbit and mouse) or are from different antibody subclasses (immunoglobulins – IgM, IgG or IgA) so that they can be distinguished by differentially labelled secondary antibodies. In this way a nuclear antigen could be labelled red, while a microtubule antigen is labelled green. Such gross subcellular distinctions can also be made using immu-nohistochemistry, but by using immunofluorescence antigens occupying virtually the same site can be identified, as the colours produced may overlap to give the impression of a third colour, which makes colocalisa-tion of different antigenic targets easy to spot. This may sound like fun (and it produces very impressive pictures), but the sting in the tail is that a UV microscope will cost much more to purchase and to maintain than a light microscope. An example of immunofluorescence in action is shown in Figure 8.1 (*see* plate section).

In situ hybridisation

In situ hybridisation is a system for detecting the presence of DNA and RNA in both histological and cytological preparations. Essentially as in Southern and/or northern blotting, the method relies on the fact that complementary nucleotide sequences will hybridise together. However, the main advantage of *in situ* hybridisation over these related techniques is that it allows for the specific cells containing the nucleic acids of interest to be visualised. Hence by using labelled nucleic acid sequences as probes complementary to the sequence of interest, both the existence *and* the position of the target can be verified.

In situ hybridisation has a variety of different applications. One of these is looking at gene expression which allows you to study the phenotype of particular cells. It may also be used to target viral transcripts, which will identify infected cells. In addition, DNA *in situ* hybridisation can be used to identify the presence of viral genomes, and for studying the karyotype of a cell.

Of course choosing the right probe is very important. Probes can be made from either DNA or RNA, depending on the application and the nature of the target. You can target both DNA and RNA with either type of probe, and each has its own advantages. DNA probes remain stable over long periods of time (months to years), unlike their more labile RNA counterparts. However RNA probes hybridise more efficiently than DNA probes to RNA target sequences.

To generate RNA probes, the nucleic acid sequence of interest is often cloned into an *in vitro* expression vector. This is then incubated with RNA polymerase and ribonucleotides to allow the probe to be generated via transcription. The label of choice is then incorporated during this step. One of the ribonucleotides used can be radiolabelled (e.g. S^{35}) or it can be conjugated with a fluorescent or epitope tag (e.g. FITC or digoxigenin respectively).[1]

DNA probes can come in many guises; PCR products, oligonucleotides, or cloned DNA in vectors (e.g. plasmids, cosmids), and can be labelled with 'hot' or 'cold' tags via a range of techniques. There are many proprietary kits on the market that you can use to do this, and again your lab will probably have a favoured method. An example of an *in situ* hybridisation is shown in Figure 8.2 (*see* plate section).

Reference

1   Roche, Introduction to Hapten Labeling and Detection of Nucleic Acids www.roche-applied-science.com/PROD_INF/MANUALS/InSitu/pdf/ISH_11–14.pdf

Chapter 9

Cell culture

Co-written with Dr Angelo Agathanggelou.

Principle of techniques

Cultured cells are often used in experiments as a surrogate for animals, and/or to simplify the system being studied. Thus they give a researcher a model for the whole animal, which is easier to manipulate on many levels (it doesn't matter how many cells you kill) and is on the whole much cheaper. However using this kind of 'simplified model' may mean that you don't get to see the full story.

The cells used can be of animal or human origin and can be derived from almost any tissue type. Cell lines can be obtained from many sources such as large cell repositories (for example the ATCC – American Type Culture Collection[1]) or biomedical suppliers, and are often passed around from lab to lab and traded for favours! In fact you can even set up your own from fresh tissues.

Growing cells in culture

All cell lines are different, and will have different requirements in order for them to grow. There are many different kinds of growth media available commercially, which contain various combinations of nutrients, e.g. DMEM (Dulbecco's Modified Eagle's Medium). The medium is usually supplemented with serum (e.g. FCS: fetal calf serum) that contains additional nutrients and growth factors, which help the cells to thrive and proliferate.

With all these nice things in the flask with the cells, there is an ever-present threat of invasion by microbial organisms, such as bacteria, fungi or yeast. Thus all of the handling of your cells has to be conducted in such a way as to minimise the opportunity for these 'bugs' to get in and take over! This is called working with aseptic technique and consists of using sterile plastic/glassware, handling open flasks within a sterile atmosphere created by a flow cabinet, wearing appropriate gloves and usually

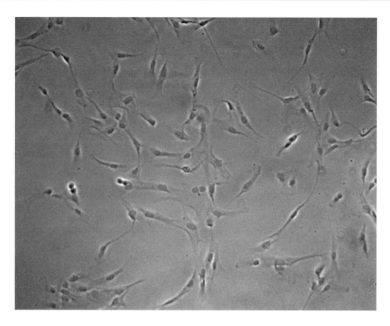

Figure 9.1 Example of cells in culture. The figure shows a phase contrast image (× 100) of adherent hTERT-RPE1 cells in culture. (Image supplied courtesy of Dr Angelo Agathanggelou, Chromatin and Gene Expression Group, Division of Immunology and Infection, University of Birmingham.)

separate lab coats which are not worn in the open lab, and not coughing on your cells . . . . To minimise this threat further, the medium is often supplemented with antibiotics e.g. pen/strep (penicillin plus streptomycin).

As the cells all originally derived from living animals, they grow best at body temperature and so are kept in incubators, usually at 37°C. In order to maintain the correct pH, the incubator atmosphere is maintained at a level of 5% CO_2. Cells that are growing well will soon reach the point where there isn't enough room for them all, and they need to be 'split'. This is called passaging and involves removing a proportion of the cells from the flask and refeeding the remainder so that they can continue to grow optimally. The removed cells can be used for an experiment, seeded into another flask to produce more cells, or discarded.

Anything that has been in contact with the cells or the medium that they were grown in must be disposed of in specific ways, determined by your lab's health and safety policy. This usually involves a sterilisation step such as autoclaving or chemical treatments (e.g. Virkon), and is often followed by incineration.

Primary cell cultures

Cells that are derived from fresh tissues and grown in flasks essentially unchanged are called primary cultures. These are normal cells, and so are only capable of a certain number of cell divisions before they senesce: exactly as they would have done in the whole animal. Hence it is important to keep track of the passage number because this determines how 'old' the cells are and may have an impact on your experiments. Examples of primary cultures are HUVECs (human umbilical venous epithelial cells) and MEFs (mouse embryonal fibroblasts).

To overcome this problem of limited proliferative capacity, cells can be immortalised. This can be achieved by transfecting the cells with telomerase, which will ensure that the telomeres are not eroded during cell division, and hence the cells will not senesce and will proliferate indefinitely.

Transformed cell cultures

Many cell lines are derived from tumours that grow well in culture by virtue of the fact that they are already immortalised as part of the transformation process inherent in tumorigenesis. Like cells immortalised using telomerase, cell lines derived from tumours often proliferate rapidly and need to be split regularly.

Transformed cells differ from immortalised cells in that they are not subject to contact inhibition, have reduced serum dependence, exhibit anchorage-independent growth and can produce tumours when injected into athymic (nude) mice.

What can you do with your cell culture? You can use the cells to test the effects of various drugs or toxins, infect them with viruses or introduce new genes to exogenously express a particular protein of interest. You can even knockdown the activity of a gene by introducing siRNA (small inhibitory RNA).

This is by no means an exhaustive list: the potential applications for cell lines in biomedical research are vast and are always growing. With so many possibilities, choosing the best cell line for your investigation is obviously very important. For example, if you were interested in breast cancer, then you would use a cell line derived from a breast tumour to work with. Not all cell lines are amenable to all manipulation techniques, and so choosing the right one from the plethora of options is crucial to your experimental outcomes.

Examples of common cell lines you may encounter include 3T3 mouse fibroblast cells, HEK293 (human embryonic kidney) cells and the famous HeLa (Henrietta Lacks) cervical carcinoma cell line, which has been growing in thousands of labs worldwide for decades. In 1951 Henrietta Lacks was diagnosed with cervical cancer, and samples of her cells were grown in culture and survived very well.[2,3] Since then they have been grown as an unbroken line and used for much of the basic work on cell physiology. The cells are all now very different from each other (probably) due to mutations and different growth environments.

This is an important point: transformed cells are by their very nature *different* from normal cells and you must not lose sight of this when interpreting any data you produce from them.

References

1   American Type Culture Collection. www.lgcpromochem-atcc.com/ (accessed 27 June 2006).
2   Disenchanted Dictionary – *Helacyton gartleri*. www.disenchanted.com/dis/ lookup. html?node=1860 (accessed 27 June 2006).
3   Cavanagh T. Where can I find out more about HeLa cells? www.madsci.org/ posts/ archives/may97/860431113.Cb.r.html (accessed 27 June 2006).

Chapter 10

Molecular biology

Co-written with Dr Angelo Agathanggelou.

Introduction to molecular biology

The basic concept of molecular biology is to investigate the activities of an organism's makeup at a subcellular level. Thus the focus is on the sequence of the DNA, the genes, the rate and timing of the expression of those genes, the mechanisms involved in expressing those genes, and the effect that they have on the whole cell and ultimately the whole organism. Many different techniques have developed to help researchers unpack these complex processes, in order to understand better the mechanisms and perhaps to exploit them as therapeutics in the fight against disease. This chapter will attempt to introduce the basic concepts of some of the most common techniques, and will explain what each technique can be used for, what it can tell, and, perhaps more importantly, what it can't!

Southern blotting

Nucleic-acid blotting techniques are very similar in principle. The idea is that a piece of DNA of interest is cut up into fragments, separated out on a gel and then the fragments are blotted onto the surface of a solid membrane. Once here they can be probed with a complementary sequence that has some kind of marker, which we can see and measure. Thus the presence of a particular sequence of DNA can be studied. The first technique of this kind, looking at DNA fragments and using single-stranded DNA as a probe, was described by Ed Southern in 1975 and quickly acquired the nickname 'Southern blotting'.[1]

In Southern blotting, genomic DNA is extracted from cells and is 'digested' using restriction enzymes. These are enzymes that very specifically cleave DNA only at particular palindromic sequences, leaving either blunt or overhanging (sticky) ends. Thus a length of DNA if digested by, for example, *Eco*R1 will only be cut at sections with the sequence:

5'-G ✂ AATTC-3'
3'-CTTAA ✂ G-5'

By using different restriction enzymes, with different cleavage sites, there is a great range of restriction fragments that can be produced. There are many restriction enzymes commercially available, and they can be chosen according to need, to cut at either a commonly found or more rarely seen sequence.

Once the DNA has been reduced, the fragments can be separated according to size via electrophoresis on an agarose gel. Care must be taken to ensure that the DNA does not hybridise to itself, but remains as single-stranded fragments. Usually separation occurs in a horizontal tank, and the agarose gel is often made up containing ethidium bromide. This carcinogenic compound intercalates with the DNA (hence its carcinogenic properties) and means that when illuminated with a UV light, the fragments can be seen, and the progress of the separation judged. As ethidium bromide is such a nasty chemical to handle and dispose of, there are more pleasant alternatives on the market such as SYB green, but these often have inherent difficulties of their own, such as a reduction in resolution. Each lab generally has a favoured way of visualising DNA in gels, which may depend on what will happen to the fragments in the next stage of the protocol. If visualisation itself was the object of the gel being run, then once a photograph/scan is taken, the gel will be discarded. However if the DNA is then blotted and probed, molecules such as ethidium bromide can interfere. A way around this is to run multiple lanes on a gel, and the outer one is removed and stained to check for good separation. It is reasonable to assume that the other lanes have run in a similar fashion, and these can then proceed onto the next stage.

The separated DNA fragments are then transferred or blotted onto a nylon (or sometimes nitrocellulose) membrane to hold them static and make them robust enough to be handled and probed. The simplest way of blotting DNA is via capillary blotting where a sandwich is made by the gel, the membrane and dry filter paper. The stack is placed in a reservoir of buffer, which is drawn through the gel and membrane into the dry paper by capillary action. The movement of the buffer takes the DNA fragments out of the gel and into the membrane, where they can be fixed by baking or exposure to UV light which cross-links the DNA. Figure 10.1 shows a schematic for the Southern blotting protocol, and Figure 10.2 illustrates a common simple method for a capillary blotting set-up.

Once firmly fixed to the membrane, the DNA fragments can be subjected to multiple rounds of probing and washes without loss of sample, as long as care is taken to maintain the pH of the solutions and the stringency

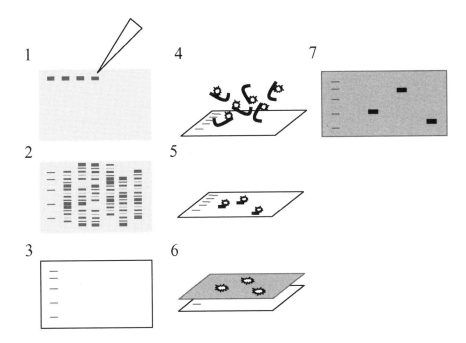

Figure 10.1 Illustration of a basic Southern blotting protocol showing: (1) loading of the prepared DNA sample into the wells of the agarose gel; (2) separation of the DNA after electrophoresis. Bands are illustrative only – you would only see the dye front, unless ethidium bromide is included and the gel is viewed under UV light; (3) separated DNA is transferred onto a nylon membrane by capillary blotting (*see* Figure 10.2); (4) in the hybridisation step, labelled probe is applied to the membrane; (5) the labelled probe hybridises to the sections of DNA that have a complementary sequence; (6) the membrane is exposed to hyperfilm, which reacts to the light or the radioactivity to produce a band; (7) the hyperfilm shows dark patches, which correspond to the target DNA.

of the washes. Stringency is an important consideration, and we will come back to it later.

One of the most complex considerations of using this technique is the construction of an appropriate probe. A lot of thought must be given to what exactly it is that you are trying to find out, and what kind of probe is going to give you that information. Put simply, a probe is a short sequence of DNA that you have chosen or designed because it is complementary to the sequence of genomic DNA you are interested in. Thus great care must be taken not to muddle coding and non-coding strands, or get the sequences back to front! Let us imagine that we want to know if gene X is present on a piece of extracted DNA. We know the sequence of gene X and can therefore design a short primer sequence that is complementary

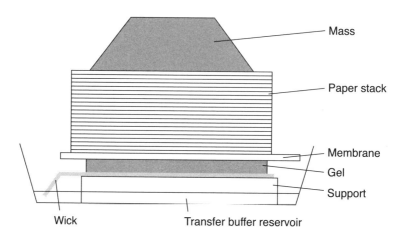

Figure 10.2 Capillary transfer set-up. The classic set-up uses the capillary forces of a buffer being drawn up a wick through the gel and membrane into a stack of tissues. The mass on the top helps to reduce the possibility of air bubbles existing between the gel and the membrane, and draws the buffer up to the tissue stack. The transfer may take a few hours but must be standardised for each protocol. Alternative set-ups are available, including using a gentle vacuum pump to transfer the DNA.

to it. The next step is to construct a probe to our design, and attach to it some kind of recognition system. A common system, although one not without inherent hazards, is to use radiolabelling. In this way a base with a radioactive tag (often P^{32} or S^{35}) is used to make the probe. Thus wherever this 'hot' piece of DNA goes, we can find it by measuring its radioactive signal. Obviously care must be taken when making and handling these probes, and there are problems with decay rates and sensitivities. Again alternative methods are available where other molecules are used to tag the DNA, which are then identified using antibodies, conjugated to enzymes, which produce a small amount of light. While safer to use, these 'cold' systems can sometimes be more complex and may have a reduced sensitivity. Again, each lab tends to have its own favoured method.

Whichever system is used, the next step is to introduce the labelled probe to the membrane which has the target DNA fixed to it. This is the hybridisation step, and it is very important that the conditions chosen are correct for the probe you are using and the target you are looking for. Non-specific binding of the probe to any old bit of DNA, or the membrane itself, must be kept to a minimum, while the amount of binding to the target is maximised. Thus a fair amount of tinkering with solutions and temperatures is often needed before the ideal set of conditions is found. This is where stringency comes in!

Stringency is determined by the salt concentration and the temperature of your wash buffers. DNA hybridisation is more favourable under high-salt/low-temperature conditions, but this means that you may risk increasing the level of non-specific binding. Stringency of binding increases with higher temperature and lower salt; in other words under these conditions only interactions between exactly complementary sequences may occur, which reduces the level of non-specific binding. However if your stringency is too high you may strip your probe straight off again!

After hybridisation of the probe to the target, the membrane is washed to remove any non-bound probe and then is exposed to a sensitive type of photographic film. The areas where the probe has bound, and where the target DNA is to be found, will produce a dark exposed section on the film (whether the probe is hot or chemiluminescent). Thus the existence (and size) of the target DNA is confirmed. By using different restriction enzymes this technique can be used to map sequences around interesting genes.

Northern blotting

This type of nucleic acid blotting is similar to Southern blotting, but instead of targeting DNA, the molecule of interest is RNA. Nicknamed 'northern blotting', the technique uses exactly the same principle of separating the RNA by running out the sample on a horizontal gel, before transferring it to a nylon membrane for probing with a homologous DNA probe. However the different nature of the RNA molecule compared to a DNA molecule means that a very different handling technique and a different environment is required.

Northern blotting is often used to discover if the RNA for a particular gene is present in a particular cell. DNA may well be the master copy of the information to make an organism, but unless a particular gene is being expressed (first by making RNA, and then ultimately the protein for which that gene codes), then the cell isn't 'using' that gene. Measuring the levels of RNA for a specific gene can give you a good indication of the level of expression of that gene, and a possible hint at the potential protein levels. Unlike DNA, which is pretty tough, RNA is a much more fragile, heat labile, fall apart as soon as you look at it kind of molecule. Thus much of the detail of the northern method is concerned with preserving the

RNA as much as possible, so as to result in a representative value for the RNA levels in a particular cell.

RNA is degraded by RNAses, so you must be aware of the precautions taken to reduce the chances of this occurring. As RNAses are pretty much everywhere, avoiding them involves always wearing appropriate lab coats/gloves (interestingly here you are protecting the work from you, and not the other way around!), having a designated set of pipettes which are treated and then only used for RNA work, only using 'RNAse-free' microtubes and pipette tips etc. Your lab may have a section of bench or even a small room designated for RNA work only, which helps to keep possible contamination down. RNAses can be treated by very high temperatures, for example glassware can be rendered RNAse free by baking (250–300°C for many hours), or by using chemicals. A common chemical treatment is diethylpyrocarbonate; usually abbreviated to DEPC, which cross-links and inactivates RNAses when solutions are treated, left for a few hours and then autoclaved. Many labs treat all of their distilled water used for making up all of the reagents involved in RNA work with DEPC. However DEPC is itself very nasty stuff (possibly carcinogenic), and has to be handled in a fume hood. Various companies make alternatives such as RNAZap, but as with many things your lab probably has its own preferred tried and tested method. If you want to get the best results from your RNA, you also have to consider how you are going to prepare and store it. The easiest way is probably to snap-freeze the tissue samples in liquid nitrogen, in small enough chunks to ensure immediate freezing of the whole piece. Samples can then be stored in a –80°C freezer for at least 12 months. Other methods include homgenisation with cell lysis solutions, or treatment with proprietary kits designed to preserve RNA. If you are going to be handling a lot of precious samples for a large study, it may well be worth spending some time investigating the best method for protecting, extracting and storing your RNA samples with some scrap tissue, before you start on the real thing. Intact RNA should show two clear ribosomal bands at 28 and 18S with a smear of other sizes when run out on an agarose gel. Degraded RNA will appear as a smear, usually at lower molecular weights, as the larger RNA molecules break up.[2]

The rest of the northern protocol is very similar to that of the Southern technique, consisting of transfer of the separated RNA strands onto a solid support membrane, fixing and then probing. Finally the location of the probe is visualised using the appropriate type of sensitive film. Thus Southern, northern and western blotting together make up a range of useful techniques that enable you to study DNA, RNA and protein levels in tissues.

PCR and RT-PCR

The polymerase chain reaction (PCR) is a very powerful technique that has completely opened up the field of molecular biology over the past decade or so. The beauty of the technique is its apparent simplicity. PCR basically allows you to take any piece of DNA you are interested in, be it an extract from a cancer cell, a sample from a mosquito from a piece of ancient amber(!), or blood/urine samples in the clinic, and make enough copies of it for you to work with and investigate it fully. Thus tiny fractions of genes too small to be identified by other methods can be amplified and copied *ad infinitum*, allowing you to do whatever you want with them!

The basic principle of the method exploits the fact that DNA is double-stranded, and if you denature the helix using high temperatures, you can make another complementary strand using DNA polymerase and a few loose bases, effectively doubling the amount of DNA you have. If you do that again and again, you can see how you can make lots of copies, all identical to the original strand. What makes this technique practical is the use of automation by engaging the services of the highly temperature-resistant DNA polymerase from *Thermus aquaticus*. This bacteria lives in hot springs, and is quite happy at temperatures around 100°C. Most other DNA polymerases only work at low temperatures, but DNA only denatures into two strands at high temperatures. Thus *Taq* polymerase can be used to make copies of DNA by cycling between high and low temperatures every few minutes, so in the space of a few hours you can amplify one copy of DNA up to millions! PCR machines costing a few thousand pounds are fundamentally programmable heating/cooling blocks that take your samples up and down to exact temperatures for an exact number of cycles, before cooling the amplified DNA ready for use. Many labs with high usage of PCR techniques will have banks of machines running 24 hours a day.

PCR consists of three basic steps. The first is a heating step, usually up to about 95°C for about a minute, which denatures the target DNA into single strands. The temperature is then cooled to around 50–70°C, and specially designed primers (short sections of DNA which are complementary to the target) anneal to the DNA and provide a starting point for the *Taq* polymerase. The final step is DNA synthesis (72°C), where the *Taq* generates new DNA strands using the dNTPs (deoxyribonucleotide triphosphates) provided in the mix, starting at the primers and following the original template strand (*see* Figure 10.3).

As with most molecular biology techniques, the theory is simple, but

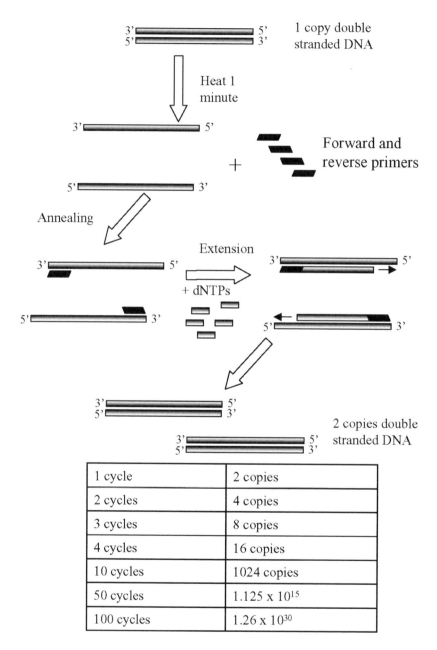

1 cycle	2 copies
2 cycles	4 copies
3 cycles	8 copies
4 cycles	16 copies
10 cycles	1024 copies
50 cycles	1.125×10^{15}
100 cycles	1.26×10^{30}

Figure 10.3 Schematic diagram showing a basic PCR reaction. Double-stranded original DNA is denatured into two strands and forward and reverse primers are annealed onto the target DNA to provide a starting point for the extension step. The *Taq* polymerase synthesises new DNA complementary to the original sequence, using dNTPs, resulting in two copies of the DNA sequence of interest. The table shows the potential power of the technique to produce multiple copies of target DNA when using a relatively small number of cycles.

actually doing it can be more problematic. PCR will amplify any piece of DNA in the mix, and so the reagents and working conditions have to be kept extremely clean and completely DNA free. This usually means a separate set of pipettes, separate working areas, DNA-free plasticware etc. Often a water control tube is included in each run. This contains no target DNA, and so if DNA appears in the mix at the end of the cycles, then you know you have a contaminated reagent. People (especially students) have been known to accidentally PCR their own DNA via sloppy technique!

Details such as choosing the correct annealing temperature for your samples, extension time, and designing your primers correctly can all contribute to the success of your PCR, as can the quantity of DNA you initially use and the concentration of magnesium in the mix. So time spent adjusting the conditions to find the optimum set for that particular target will be time well spent. PCR products are usually verified by running them out on an ethidium bromide agarose gel and checking that there is a band, and that it is the size you were expecting. Primers can sometimes fit onto other sections of the template DNA, and so you may have amplified a completely different section from that which you wanted, giving you an additional band on the gel.

RT-PCR (reverse transcription PCR) is an extension to the PCR system that allows amplification of RNA sequences. It is a much more sensitive way of studying RNA quantification than northern blotting. As *Taq* polymerase only works on DNA and won't read/copy an RNA sequence, an extra step is needed. This step uses the enzyme reverse transcriptase (RT), which makes a cDNA copy of the RNA sequence you have in your mix. The primers and dNTPs then get on with the PCR reactions as normal. The end product is a double-stranded piece of DNA, which has the same sequence as the RNA target you started with.

Real-time RT-PCR takes the level of investigation a stage further. In normal RT-PCR the reactions continue to an 'end-point' chosen by you, e.g. 30–40 cycles, and this will give you lots of product which you can then use for further experiments, e.g. cloning. However this method is not particularly quantitative. If you want to know how much RNA your samples have, e.g. if you are interested in the level of expression of a particular gene, then real-time can tell you this, as you can 'see' how much product is being produced as you go along. Real-time RT-PCR uses a fluorescent probe system, of which there are several available on the market (e.g. TaqMan, Molecular Beacons, Scorpion), which basically means that the product 'glows' and can be measured by a spectrophotometer built into the thermal cycler during the cycles occurring in the exponential phase of the amplification, which enables accurate determination of the RNA levels in your sample.[3–5]

Microarray/chip systems

Another tool recently added to the molecular biologist's kit are the microarray or chip systems. These are high-throughput technologies which allow, among other applications, global changes in gene expression to be investigated. There are various array systems but the principle by which they all work is basically the same. In northern blotting, the sample RNA is immobilised onto a membrane which is then probed by a single-labelled oligonucleotide or cDNA sequence. In microarrays it is the RNA sample that is used to generate the probe. Labelled cDNA is generated by reverse transcription incorporating a dye such as Cy3. The resulting probe is used to interrogate 'chips', often made of glass, which contain thousands of arrayed oligonucleotide or cDNA sequences. A scanner measures the amount of labelled probe bound to each arrayed nucleotide sequence. An example of a microarray is shown in Figure 10.4 (*see* plate section).

The type of array used depends on the questions that you are trying to address and often, perhaps more importantly, the budget you have available to you. Microarrays are not cheap! In general there are two types: the spotted array and the photolithographically synthesised oligonucleotide arrays. Spotted arrays are generated by, not surprisingly, a spotter which uses glass needles to deliver a very small quantity of a particular DNA sequence, e.g. cDNA, oligonucleotides or plasmids. Most institutions using microarrays will have a 'spotting machine' allowing customised arrays to be generated to order. The advantage of the spotted array is that it is relatively cheap; however it can suffer from a potential reduction in spotting quality, such as inaccuracy in spot position and uniformity.

In photolithographically generated arrays, short oligonucleotides (often 19–21mers and up to 60mers) are synthesised on the glass matrix. This allows the arrays to be produced at a much higher density of 'spots per inch' than the spotted arrays and with a far superior uniformity. This is reflected in their much higher costs, often 10× more expensive!

In addition to gene expression analysis, the high thoughput power of microarrays is used for applications such as comparative genomic hybridisation (CGH) analysis, which track global changes in genomic instability, identify novel genes, group genes into functional pathways and identify potential binding sites for transcription factors.[6]

Thus the field of microarrays research is rapidly expanding, with many new applications emerging.

Web-based resources

There are many web-based resources to help you prepare for your experiments. In fact a lot can be achieved *in silico* before you even put on a lab coat. Since the completion of the human and other genomes there is an increasing need to be computer savvy and make use of web-based programs and databases. The National Center for Biotechnology Information (NCBI) website[7] supports the GenBank DNA sequence database. Using the Entrez tool,[8] you'll be able to search and retrieve RNA, DNA and protein sequences from various organisms. In addition NCBI supports databases such as Online Mendelian Inheritance in Man (OMIM),[9] Unique Human Gene Sequence Collection (UniGene),[10] and The Cancer Genome Anatomy Project (CGAP).[11] Useful programs available on the NCBI website include BLAST,[12] which is a powerful sequence similarity searching tool for nucleotide and protein sequences, and Open Reading Frame Finder (ORF Finder).[13] For those important literature searches there's PubMed,[14] which provides access to MEDLINE,[15] and will allow you to peruse over 11 million citations.

The University of California Santa Cruz Genome Bioinformatics website contains reference sequences and draft assemblies for a large collection of organisms.[16] It is home to Genome Browser,[17] which is a very user-friendly tool that allows you to scan across chromosomes and examine the annotations provided by the scientific community.

A range of proteomics tools are available on the ExPASY (Expert Protein Analysis System) Proteomics Server.[18] This provides access to a myriad of programs for activities such as protein identification and characterisation, similarity searches, pattern and profile searches, post-translation modification prediction, topology prediction, primary structure analysis, secondary and tertiary structure analysis, sequence alignment and phylogenetic analysis.

References

1 Southern EM. Detection of specific sequences among DNA fragments separated by gel electrophoresis. *Journal of Molecular Biology* 1975; 98: 503–17.
2 Ambion. *Ten Ways to Improve Your RNA Isolation*. TechNotes 9(1). www.ambion.com/techlib/tn/91/9113.html (accessed 27 June 2006).
3 Ambion. *The Basics*. www.ambion.com/techlib/basics/index.html

4   Powledge TM. The polymerase chain reaction. www.faseb.org/opa/bloodsupply/pcr. html

5   Mama Ji's Molecular Kitchen. http://lifesciences.asu.edu/resources/mamajis/index. html (accessed 27 June 2006).

6   Stoughton RB. Applications of DNA microarrays in biology. *Annual Review of Biochemistry* 2005; 74: 53–82.

7   National Center for Biotechnology Information. www.ncbi.nih.gov/ (accessed 27 June 2006).

8   Entrez, the Life Sciences Search Engine. www.ncbi.nlm.nih.gov/gquery/gquery.fcgi (accessed 27 June 2006).

9   Online Mendelian Inheritance in Man. www.ncbi.nlm.nih.gov/entrez/query. fcgi? db=OMIM (accessed 27 June 2006).

10 Unique Human Gene Sequence Collection (UniGene). www.ncbi.nlm.nih.gov/entrez/query.fcgi?db=unigene&cmd=search&term=unigene

11 Cancer Genome Anatomy Projects. www.ncbi.nlm.nih.gov/CGAP/ (accessed 27 June 2006).

12 BLAST. www.ncbi.nlm.nih.gov/BLAST/ (accessed 27 June 2006).

13 Open Reading Frame Finder. www.ncbi.nlm.nih.gov/gorf/gorf.html (accessed 27 June 2006).

14 PubMed. www.ncbi.nlm.nih.gov/entrez/query.fcgi?db=PubMed (accessed 27 June 2006).

15 MEDLINE. http://medline.cos.com/ (accessed 27 June 2006).

16 University of California Santa Cruz Genome Bioinformatics. http://genome.ucsc.edu/ (accessed 27 June 2006).

17 Genome Browser. http://genome.ucsc.edu/cgi-bin/hgGateway (accessed 27 June 2006).

18 ExPASY. www.expasy.org/ (accessed 27 June 2006).

Chapter 11

Using animals in biomedical research

Introduction

If you are going to be involved in biomedical research it is probably inevitable that you will come across the use of animals or their tissues during the course of your experiments. This chapter is not going to examine the debate around this issue; instead it will lay out some of the basic facts about the use of animals in research and give an overview of the legislation that is in place in the UK. It is very important that you understand these regulations and that if you are involved in using animals in your research, you comply absolutely with the guidelines and the law.

Basic facts and figures

Why are animals used in biomedical research? The answer to this question is complex and varies depending on what you mean by biomedical research. A simple answer is that animals are used in research to help answer important questions that cannot be answered any other way; when it is necessary to find out what is happening in a whole living body, or in the way different body systems interact with each other under particular circumstances. Approximately 10% of biomedical research is based on the use of animals.

Obviously no researcher wishes to use animals when other methods could meet the scientific objective, and so for any new experimental plan there are three guiding principles that all researchers must adhere to. These are referred to as the Three 'Rs'. The first 'R' is *replacement*. This effectively means that using animals to answer the scientific question being asked should be the last, and not the first option. Every other possible non-animal technique should be considered and shown to be inappropriate before animal studies are chosen. Some current research is focused solely on finding and developing new non-animal techniques that other researchers can then use in their experiments. If it has been decided that the scientific question can only be answered by using animals, then the other two 'Rs' come into play. The first of these is to *reduce* the number of animals used in the experiment to the absolute minimum. This comes down (once again) to accurate planning so that the data from the experiment will be statistically viable and of a certain power. If too few animals are used, this may not be the case, and so the experiment will have been unreliable and animals will have been used unnecessarily. Worse still, the experiment may have to be repeated afresh and so those animals' lives will have been wasted. On the other hand, if too many animals are used, the results might well be OK, but some animals will have been used unnecessarily, i.e. with no gain in the scientific objective. Similarly if the other aspects of the research are not properly planned and executed, then the whole experiment may fail, and have to be repeated, increasing the number of animals required. Usually animals that are genetically very similar are used, as this reduces the variation between individuals and can also help to reduce the number of animals needed to produce useful data.

The last of the 'Rs' is to *refine* the experimental plan so that any possible pain, distress, and suffering to the animals involved is avoided, alleviated or kept to an absolute minimum. Thus the researcher must show that every aspect of the experiment is designed with the animals' welfare paramount. For example they would need to explain how they are going to use painkillers or anaesthesia to prevent suffering, or use continuous drug administration to reduce the number of times an animal is restrained and injected. Refinement also considers the treatment of the animals while not actively participating in the experiment. Thus the conditions of the animal housing facilities are very closely monitored, and appropriate enrichment of their environment is considered to be very important. This includes things like keeping social animals in groups, providing toys and bedding to nest in, and making the food provided as interesting and varied as possible.

The numbers of animals used for biomedical research in the UK has fallen by more than half over the last 30 years or so, probably due to changes in legislation and increased standards of animal welfare, and also because of the application of guidelines such as the Three 'Rs'. Procedures involving animals with genetic modifications (such as gene knockout mice) are the only types that are currently increasing in number (nearly one million in 2004), but this is a relatively new field of research. Around 87% of animals used in the UK are rats, mice and other small rodents, with fish, amphibians, reptiles and birds making up 12%. Small mammals such as farm animals and rabbits make up the other 1% in addition to other groups including purpose-bred dogs and cats, and primates such as marmosets and macaques. The use of chimpanzees and other great apes is banned in the UK.[1]

Regulation of animal research

The current UK legislation relating to the use of animals in biomedical research is the 1986 Animals (Scientific Procedures) Act.[2] This is a very strict piece of legislation that tightly controls the way living vertebrate animals are used in research, while still enabling important biomedical research to continue in a productive manner. The Act also protects one invertebrate, *Octopus vulgaris*, foetal forms more than 50% of the way through gestation, and free-living forms of amphibian, e.g. tadpoles. The law is based on the idea that the likely benefits that will be obtained from the research must far outweigh the likely 'costs' in terms of any potential animal suffering. This cost– or harm–benefit analysis must be applied before any work involving animals is allowed to begin.

The Act requires that research involving the use of animals can only take place in research institutes or companies that have a certificate of designation showing that the animal facilities including staff training and veterinary support are at appropriate standards. The Home Office must also approve the work itself through the granting of a project licence. All of the people involved with the animals, from the researchers to the animal husbandry staff, must also be shown to have received sufficient appropriate training, and have the skills and experience to look after the animals correctly. Those researchers carrying out procedures on animals must also hold a personal licence for the types of procedures they are conducting, which is required before they can be involved in any experiments. Holders of a personal licence cannot carry out any work unless they are also covered for that work by a project licence: in other words having a technique on a personal licence is not sufficient to carry out that procedure on an animal; the work must have been also approved through the granting of a project licence.

Project and personal licences are difficult to obtain and can be revoked at any time by the Home Office Inspectorate on his or her advice to the Home Secretary, e.g. if there has been a breach of the conditions attached to a licence. Licences are only granted if all of the requirements are met. These include measures previously described such as the cost–benefit analysis, using the Three 'Rs', ensuring staff have the correct skills, and that the animal-handling facilities are appropriate. Thus the nature of the legislation makes individuals and institutions responsible for making sure that the best possible practice is always adhered to. The Home Office has an Inspectorate whose members are either medics or vets and who inspect institutions on a regular basis, often without warning. They check that all the appropriate regulations are being met and they have the power to stop any animal work if they feel that the standards are not high enough.

Another layer of regulation was introduced in 1999. This is the system of local ethical review, which looks at what is happening in a particular institution. Thus the laws governing the use of animals in biomedical research are enforced in the UK at both the national and local levels. The regulations are continually reviewed, and additional policies introduced as and when they are needed.

Day-to-day use of animals

So what happens on a day-to-day basis for researchers using animals in their experiments? For a start if you are new to using animals you will be expected to attend a training course, which has been accredited by the Home Office. The level of expertise you will need to reach will depend on whether you will need to hold a personal licence, or will only be peripherally involved in the work (e.g. analysing tissues or blood samples), or whether the work does not need to be regulated as the scientific procedures do not involve any pain, suffering, distress or lasting harm. You will not be allowed to be involved in the research until you have reached the satisfactory level of training, and you have shown that you meet the standards required by the course.

If you are applying for a personal licence or are involved in the process of obtaining a project licence for a programme of research, your application will normally first have to be scrutinised by the local ethical review group/committee. Different institutions will have different arrangements, but an application may go through multiple rounds of ethical consideration and review before being submitted to the Home Office for approval. Often experienced staff from the animal facility will be able to offer advice on writing suitable applications. One of the major considerations may well be the cost of purchasing and maintaining animals in the facility. When a new grant application for research is being written, if animals are to be included in the study, then the costs, licensing and ethical implications must be considered from the outset. Using animals in a study is not something that can be tagged on at the end, or decided on a whim if other routes fail. Perhaps for this, more than any other aspect of biomedical research, appropriate planning is absolutely essential.[3]

Once you have your Home Office approval and licences in place, you will need to liaise very closely with the staff running your animal housing facilities. Some facilities have animal-breeding programmes, others buy in animals as required, but either way you will have to make detailed plans and follow specific processes to order the animals that you need, for when you need them. Moving animals between establishments is also complex and requires additional paperwork, such as health reports and export licences. Once your animals are available, the facility staff will use their expert knowledge of animal husbandry to ensure that the health and welfare of the animals is maintained at the highest level, and that all standard operating procedures are adhered to. They will be focused on making sure that the environment that the animals are kept in is as enriched as possible, and is appropriate to the scientific work, and that any pain and distress is kept to the absolute minimum.

A named animal care and welfare officer (NACWO) is appointed, who is responsible for the day-to-day care of the animals that are involved in each regulated procedure, or are being used within the establishment, e.g. breeding animals. The NACWO liaises very closely with the project licence holder on the design and progress of the experiments, and the nature of the procedures. They continually monitor the animals' welfare and will advise the researcher if they have any concerns.

In addition to the NACWO, every designated scientific procedure establishment must have a named vet who also advises on the health, care and welfare of the animals, and may be involved in any surgery and anaesthesia that may be required, and any health issues that may arise. They are also responsible for ensuring that all of the appropriate documentation and records of health etc are maintained. Thus the licensing system under the 1986 Act has multiple layers of protection in place, and relies on the team working together. This helps to ensure that the legislation is adhered to and that animals involved in essential biomedical research are treated in a humane and respectful manner, to the benefit of all.

Further information on the use of animals in research is available from the RDS (formerly Research Defence Society) and from the Home Office.

References

1   Research Defence Society. *Understanding Animal Research in Society*. www.rds-online. org.uk (accessed 27 June 2006).
2   Home Office, Science and Research, Animal Testing. www.homeoffice. gov.uk/science-research/animal-testing/?version=1 (accessed 27 June 2006).
3   Animals in Scientific Procedures. http://scienceandresearch.homeoffice. gov.uk/animal-research/ (accessed 27 June 2006).

Chapter 12

Formulae at a glance

Equations

$$moles = mass\ (g)/RFM$$
$$moles = molar\ concentration \times volume\ (l)$$
$$pH = \log_{10} 1/[H^+] = -\log_{10}[H^+]$$
$$(final\ concentration\ wanted/initial\ concentration) \times final\ volume$$
$$wanted\ (ml) = initial\ concentration\ needed\ (ml)$$

Metric system multiples

Factor	Prefix	Symbol
10^{-15}	femto	f
10^{-12}	pico	p
10^{-9}	nano	n
10^{-6}	micro	μ
10^{-3}	milli	m
10^{-2}	centi	c
10^{-1}	deci	d
10	deca	da
10^2	hecto	h
10^3	kilo	k
10^6	mega	M
10^9	giga	G
10^{12}	tera	T
10^{15}	peta	P

Index